Color Atlas & Synopsis of
Sexually Transmitted Diseases

Notice

Color Atlas & Synopsis of Sexually Transmitted Diseases

THIRD EDITION

H. Hunter Handsfield, MD

Clinical Professor of Medicine
University of Washington Center for AIDS and STD
Senior Research Leader
Battelle Centers for Public Health Research and Evaluation
Seattle, Washington

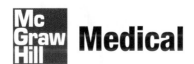

New York   Chicago   San Francisco   Lisbon   London   Madrid   Mexico City
Milan   New Delhi   San Juan   Seoul   Singapore   Sydney   Toronto

Color Atlas & Synopsis of Sexually Transmitted Diseases, Third Edition

1 2 3 4 5 6 7 8 9 10 CTP/CTP   14 13 12 11

ISBN 978-0-07-162437-4
MHID 0-07-162437-6

This book was set in Berkeley Book by Glyph International Ltd.
The editors were James Shanahan and Christie Naglieri.
The production supervisor was Sherri Souffrance.
Project management was provided by Anupriya Tyagi, Glyph International.
The designer was Mary McKeon; the cover design was by Pehrsson Design.
China Translation & Printing, Ltd. was printer and binder.

Library of Congress Cataloging-in-Publication Data

Handsfield, H. Hunter.
    Color atlas and synopsis of sexually transmitted diseases / by H. Hunter
Handsfield.—3rd ed.
        p. ; cm.
    Includes bibliographical references and index.
    ISBN-13: 978-0-07-162437-4 (pbk.)
    ISBN-10: 0-07-162437-6 (pbk.)
        1. Sexually transmitted diseases—Atlases. 2. Sexually transmitted diseases—Outlines,
syllabi, etc. I. Title.
        [DNLM: 1. Sexually Transmitted Diseases—Atlases. WC 17]
    RC200.H36 2011
    616.95'1—dc22
                                                                        2010041685

INTERNATIONAL EDITION MHID: 0-07-176818-1; ISBN: 978-0-07-176818-4

McGraw-Hill books are available at special quantity discounts to use as premiums and sales promotions, or for use in corporate training programs. To contact a representative please e-mail us at bulksales@mcgraw-hill.com.

For Evan, Nate, and Rowan

Contents

Contributors

Laura Sangaré, PhD, MPH
Senior Fellow
Department of Global Health
University of Washington
Seattle, Washington
Chapter 2: Global Epidemiology,
Prevention and Management of Sexually
Transmitted Diseases

Judd L. Walson, MD, MPH
Assistant Professor
Departments of Global Health,
Medicine (Infectious Disease),
Pediatrics, and Epidemiology
University of Washington
Seattle, Washington
Chapter 2: Global Epidemiology,
Prevention and Management of Sexually
Transmitted Diseases

Preface

Sexually transmitted diseases (STDs) are among the most common afflictions in most societie. Awareness of STDs, including HIV infection and AIDS, is high among young people in all industrialized countries and among most health care providers, a welcome change over the two decades since the first edition of this book was published. However, the general awareness by clinicians and at-risk populations does not consistently translate into accurate knowledge or clinical practice. Many young people have serious misunderstandings about STDs, with both denial by some at obvious risk and inflated fear of contagion by others. Almost all clinicians now can list *Chlamydia trachomatis* and human papillomavirus as sexually transmitted pathogens, yet STD screening is undertaken far less frequently than recommended. The vaccines against STDs are underutilized, treatment often is inconsistent with authoritative guidelines, and partners of infected persons often go untreated. This is understandable; most clinicians receive little training in STD management, and even training in HIV/AIDS often is insufficient. Further, despite the high frequency of STDs, they are not so common that most providers see infected patients daily. Except in selected settings like reproductive health, student health, and STD clinics, most patients seemingly are not at high risk and STDs are diagnosed with modest frequency.

Color Atlas and Synopsis of Sexually Transmitted Diseases is designed primarily for clinicians who find themselves caring for patients with STD or at risk, sometimes to their surprise, and need an easy-to-use aid to diagnosis, treatment, and prevention. At the same time, it contains sufficient detail to be useful for continuing education and review by highly experienced clinicians. The clinical and diagnostic procedures described are within the capabilities of the basically trained clinician and most medical offices and laboratories in industrialized countries. The epidemiologic emphasis and treatment recommendations are primarily those current in the United States, but for this edition every chapter has been modified to enhance its utility in developing countries and other resource-limited settings, and a new chapter reviews the global epidemiology of STDs. I have attempted to integrate the atlas components with the synopsis and to strike a balance between them, and users are encouraged not only to examine the photographs but to read the text and case histories. Indeed, one clinical chapter has no photographs at all. This book also can serve as a visual aid in counseling patients and will be useful to many health educators, clinic managers, and health administrators. Finally, our patients participate much more actively in their care than in the past, and the worldwide revolution in information technology has dramatically enhanced many persons' access to technical information and their ability to assimilate it. With these trends in mind, this book also is designed in part for persons with STDs or at risk, many of whom will find it useful in understanding their own infections, assessing their risk, or judging the importance of symptoms that may require clinical assessment.

The case histories are real, although some are composites of two or more patients. Most of the photographs illustrate the patients described, but some were matched with other patients whose histories were better known. For several cases from past years, the tests performed or treatments given have been updated to conform with current recommendations. The text of all chapters has been extensively rewritten to incorporate changes in epidemiology, diagnosis, and treatment since the previous edition, and the chapter on HIV infection has been greatly expanded. About a quarter of the photographs are new, and almost all the Suggested Reading citations are new and recent.

As for most books, this one has been aided by generous professional and personal support from numerous colleagues. The many who contributed clinical photographs are acknowledged in the legends; I thank them very much. My own collection of photographs began almost four decades ago and the provenance of some is uncertain; I apologize to the owners if some are not properly credited. Special thanks are due to colleagues who reviewed drafts, served as sounding boards on controversial topics, or supported me in important ways throughout my career. These include King Holmes, Larry Corey, Ned Hook, Matt Golden, Jeanne Marrazzo, Connie Celum, Sevgi Aral, Sheila Lukehart, Bob Wood, Bob Harrington, and not least Walt Stamm, whose untimely demise was a tragic loss for our field and a source of continuing sadness. Judd Walson and Laura Sangaré lent their expertise to write the new chapter on global health aspects of STDs. My editor, Jim Shanahan, remained a gentleman through all his prodding over my tardiness in getting to work on this edition, and Christie Naglieri expertly handled all the production details. Finally, I thank my wife, Patricia McInturff, for her love and support.

H. Hunter Handsfield, MD
Seattle, Washington

List of Abbreviations

AGUS	atypical glandular cells of undetermined significance
AIDS	acquired immunodeficiency syndrome
AIN	anal intraepithelial neoplasia
ARS	acute retroviral syndrome
ART	antiretroviral therapy
ARV	antiretroviral [drug]
ASCUS	atypical squamous cells of undetermined significance
bid	twice a day
BV	bacterial vaginosis
BVAB	bacterial vaginosis associated bacteria
CBC	complete blood count
CDC	Centers for Disease Control and Prevention
CMV	cytomegalovirus
CRP	C-reactive protein
CSF	cerebrospinal fluid
CSW	commercial sex worker
DALYs	disability-adjusted life years
DGI	disseminated gonococcal infection
DNA	deoxyribonucleic acid
EBV	Epstein-Barr virus
EIA	enzyme immunoassay
ELISA	enzyme-linked immunosorbent assay
EPT	expedited partner therapy
ESR	erythrocyte sedimentation rate
FTA-ABS	fluorescent treponemal antibody-absorbed test
GND	gram-negative diplococci
GUD	genital ulcer disease
HAV	hepatitis A virus
HBsAg	Hepatitis B surface antigen
HBV	hepatitis B virus
HCV	hepatitis C virus
HDV	hepatitis D virus

HHV-8	human herpesvirus 8
HIV	human immunodeficiency virus
HLA	histocompatibility locus A
HPV	human papillomavirus
HSIL	high-grade squamous intraepithelial lesion
HSV	herpes simplex virus
HTLV	human T-cell lymphotropic virus
ICGND	intracellular gram-negative diplococci
IDU	injection drug use/user
IgG	immunoglobulin G
IgM	immunoglobulin M
IM	intramuscularly
IUD	intrauterine device
IV	intravenously
LGV	lymphogranuloma venereum
LSIL	low-grade squamous intraepithelial lesion
MCV	molluscum contagiosum virus
MHA-TP	microhemagglutination assay for *Treponema pallidum*
MPC	mucopurulent cervicitis
MSM	men who have sex with men
NAAT	nucleic acid amplification test
NGU	nongonococcal urethritis
NSU	nonspecific urethritis
OHL	oral hairy leukoplakia
PCR	polymerase chain reaction
PDPT	patient-delivered partner therapy
PEP	post-exposure prophylaxis
PID	pelvic inflammatory disease
PIN	penile intraepithelial neoplasia
PITC	provider-initiated testing and counseling
PMN	polymorphonuclear [leukocyte]
PO	orally, by mouth
PrEP	pre-exposure prophylaxis
qid	four times a day
RNA	ribonucleic acid
RPR	rapid plasma reagin test
SDA	strand displacement assay
STD	sexually transmitted disease
STI	sexually transmitted infection
tid	three times a day

TMA	transcription-mediated amplification
TPHA	*Treponema pallidum* hemagglutination test
TPPA	*Treponema pallidum* particle agglutination test
TRUST	toluidine red unheated serum reagin test
UTI	urinary tract infection
VaIN	vaginal intraepithelial neoplasia
VD	venereal disease
VDRL	Venereal Disease Research Laboratory test
VIN	vulvar intraepithelial neoplasia
VVC	vulvovaginal candidiasis
WBC	white blood cell [count]
WHO	World Health Organization
WSW	women who have sex with women

• Section One

Overview of Sexually Transmitted Diseases

1

Clinical Approach to Patients with STDs or at Risk

INTRODUCTION

In few areas of infectious diseases have changes in epidemiology and our understanding of clinical manifestations been as profound as in the field of sexually transmitted diseases (STDs) during the past four decades. Sexually transmitted diseases embody all the elements of emerging infections, with continuing recognition of apparently new pathogens, syndromes, and complications; emergence of antimicrobial resistance in some pathogens; rising importance and improved understanding of viral infections; the dominant influence of demography and behavior over technological advances such as improved diagnosis and treatment; and rapid international spread fostered by the worldwide revolution in travel, population migration, commerce, and communication technologies.

Women are selectively and more seriously affected than men by almost all STDs. Many of them are transmitted more efficiently from men to women than the reverse, because the vagina serves as a reservoir that prolongs exposure to partners' genital secretions, and the female genital tract is comprised of more susceptible, noncornified epithelium. Women are more likely to have subclinical or entirely asymptomatic infections, and the diagnosis of some STDs and other genital syndromes is more difficult than in men. Most important, anatomic and physiologic conditions render women at greater risk than men for long-lasting or permanent sequelae, such as cancer, infertility, and adverse outcomes of pregnancy.

Most persons are at substantial risk for STD during their teen and young adult years. At least 80% of sexually active persons acquire one or more genital human papillomavirus (HPV) infections during their sexually active years; 50% become infected within their first three or four lifetime sex partners. More than 15% of the U.S. population, and at least 50% in some countries, acquire genital herpes simplex virus type 2 (HSV-2) infection by age 40. And each year 6 million and 3 million persons in the United States are estimated to acquire trichomoniasis and genital *Chlamydia trachomatis* infection, respectively, and the rates probably are equivalent in most other countries. Complications of STDs continue to occur for years after adoption of lower-risk lifestyles, and almost all primary care clinicians and many specialists regularly provide care to patients with STDs or their sequelae.

As for all medical conditions, clinical recognition and diagnosis of STDs are central to treatment and prevention, and these are the focus of this book. This chapter presents an overview of the clinical approach to STD diagnosis and management. The emphasis is on etiologic management, assuming availability of modern diagnostic and screening technologies and, for readily treated conditions, unrestricted access to effective therapy. Chapter 2 addresses the epidemiology and management of STDs in resource-poor settings, such as developing countries.

TERMINOLOGY

Over the years, medical and social considerations have fostered changes in the language used to characterize infections associated with sexual activity. Venereal disease (VD) was the nearly universal inclusive term through the 1960s, and referred more or less exclusively to five infections: syphilis, gonorrhea, lymphogranuloma venereum, chancroid, and donovanosis (granuloma inguinale). Other genital syndromes like nongonococcal urethritis, trichomoniasis, and genital warts and herpes were understood by dermatovenereologists and other experts to be associated with sexual activity, albeit sometimes with ingenious and even ludicrous explanations why they were not in fact sexually transmitted. When evolving research documented sexual transmission, these and other syndromes were not "VD" as historically defined. Further, VD gained increasingly pejorative connotations as the emerging infections were increasingly recognized to be prevalent in the "general population"—a euphemism for people presumably more responsible in their sexuality than those with syphilis or gonorrhea. Thus was born "sexually transmitted diseases," or STD.

The 1990s saw increasing use of "sexually transmitted infections," or STI. It was increasingly recognized that many such infections are entirely asymptomatic or cause only mild or trivial symptoms easily ignored or disregarded by patients and clinicians alike. Some subclinical infections, especially genital infections with HPV and HSV, seemed to carry few serious health implications. Such conditions, it was reasoned, are infections but not "diseases." Even asymptomatic infection with human immunodeficiency virus (HIV) was widely regarded as distinct from overt AIDS, and it was common to inform patients that they did not have AIDS, but "only" infection with HIV. Additionally, some prevention experts and patient advocates came to believe "disease" to be more pejorative than "infection" and began to view "STD" in a similar light as "VD." Still more recently, however, evolved scientific understanding has undercut the first rationale. Most infections, including those caused by HSV and HPV, have potentially serious outcomes whether symptomatic or subclinical, and without treatment asymptomatic HIV infection progresses to AIDS and nearly always to a fatal outcome. Arguably, therefore, the distinction between "infection" and "disease" is moot. Further, there is room for debate about differing connotations of the two words. Few qualitative research studies, if any, have documented that infected persons in fact interpret the terms differently.

Today, STD and STI both remain in common use. The American Sexually Transmitted Diseases Association (which originated as the American VD Association) retains its current name, its journal remains *Sexually Transmitted Diseases*, and the Centers for Disease Control and Prevention (CDC) division responsible for national prevention strategies remains the Division of STD Prevention. On the other hand, the

British Journal of Venereal Diseases changed to *Sexually Transmitted Infections*, the venerable International Union against Venereal Diseases and Treponematoses became the International Union against STI, and the World Health Organization prefers STI over STD. Consistent with dominant usage in the United States, in its third edition this book retains its original title. Today there is little or no difference in meaning by most users and the two terms should be considered synonymous.

CLASSIFICATION OF STDs

Sexually transmitted diseases can be classified according to the causative pathogens (see Table 1–1). However, many STD syndromes are caused by more than one pathogen, and nonsexually transmitted agents often contribute to pathogenesis. Table 1–2 lists the major STD clinical syndromes and sequelae in order of their public health importance. (Note that the first half of Table 1–2 is dominated by syndromes that predominantly affect women and children.) Both the etiologic and syndromic organizations are used in this book.

Table 1–1 SEXUALLY TRANSMITTED PATHOGENS

Bacteria	Viruses
Chlamydia trachomatis	Human immunodeficiency virus, types 1 and 2
Neisseria gonorrhoeae	Herpes simplex virus, types 1 and 2
Treponema pallidum	Human papillomavirus, many types
Haemophilus ducreyi	Hepatitis viruses A, B, C, and D
Calymmatobacterium granulomatis	Cytomegalovirus
Ureaplasma urealyticum	Epstein-Barr virus
Mycoplasma genitalium	Human herpesvirus type 8[+]
Salmonella species	Molluscum contagiosum virus
Shigella species	Enteric viruses
Campylobacter species	
Other enteric bacteria	
Sexually transmitted bacteria of uncertain pathogenicity[*]	

Protozoa	Ectoparasites
Trichomonas vaginalis	*Phthirus pubis* (pubic louse)
Entamoeba histolytica	*Sarcoptes scabiei* (scabies mite)
Giardia lamblia	
Other enteric protozoa	

[*]Several bacteria found in the genital tract may be shared between sex partners, but their contributions to clinical morbidity or the importance of sexual transmission are uncertain. Examples include *Mycoplasma hominis*, *Ureaplasma parvum* (formerly not distinguished from *U. urealyticum*), *Gardnerella vaginalis*, *Mobiluncus* species, group B *Streptococcus*, and bacterial vaginosis associated bacteria (BVAB) types 1–3. The contribution of sexual transmission to colonization with the yeasts *Candida albicans* and *C. glabrata* is unclear.

[+]HHV-8 is also known as Kaposi sarcoma herpes virus.

Table 1–2 MAJOR STD CLINICAL SYNDROMES AND COMPLICATIONS

1. Acquired immunodeficiency syndrome (AIDS)
2. Pelvic inflammatory disease
3. Female infertility and ectopic pregnancy
4. Fetal and neonatal infections: conjunctivitis, pneumonia, pharyngeal infection, encephalitis, neurological deficits, cognitive impairment, immunodeficiency
5. Complications of pregnancy and delivery: spontaneous abortion, premature labor, premature rupture of fetal membranes, chorioamnionitis, postpartum endometritis
6. Neoplasia: cervical dysplasia and carcinoma, Kaposi sarcoma, hepatocellular carcinoma, squamous cell carcinomas of anus, vulva, and penis
7. Human papillomavirus infection and genital warts
8. Genital ulcer—inguinal lymphadenopathy
9. Lower genital tract infection in women: cervicitis, urethritis, vaginal infection
10. Urethritis in men
11. Viral hepatitis
12. Neurosyphilis and tertiary syphilis
13. Epididymitis
14. Gastrointestinal infections: proctitis, enteritis, colitis
15. Acute arthritis
16. Mononucleosis
17. Molluscum contagiosum
18. Ectoparasite infestation

POPULATIONS AT RISK: CORE GROUPS AND SEXUAL NETWORKS

Recognition of the social and demographic markers for STD is the first step in risk assessment and clinical management. Persistence of an STD in a population is determined by complex interactions between the pathogens, the course of infection with and without treatment, and sexual behavior. Subpopulations thought to be critical to sustain the infection, and which serve as bridges of transmission to the wider population, have been termed *core groups*. Typically, core groups were defined by number of sex partners, frequency of recurrent STD, and similar factors. In recent years, the development of dynamic models of STD transmission has helped shift the epidemiologic focus to *sexual networks*, consisted of both core transmitters and other persons whose behavior patterns are conducive to STD spread.

Gonorrhea is transmitted with high efficiency; each sexual exposure between an infected and susceptible partner carries a high probability of transmission. However, gonorrhea usually is transmissible for a relatively brief period of time, typically a few days to weeks, because early symptoms result in prompt care and treatment. Accordingly, propagation of infection depends on infected persons having new sex partners soon after acquisition, which in turn requires high rates of partner change in the population at risk. By contrast, genital HSV and HPV infections persist and are transmissible for months or years, often by persons who remain unaware of their infections, so that low rates of partner change—rates that are typical throughout most populations—are sufficient to sustain transmission. Therefore, in industrialized countries gonorrhea tends to be concentrated in small subsets of the population that have especially high rates of partner change, often characterized by poverty, poor access to health care, substance abuse, and social disruption, including war and population migration—i.e., classically defined core groups. By contrast, genital herpes and HPV infections are common in all segments of society, including persons often considered at low risk. Chlamydial infection occupies an intermediate position. It causes largely asymptomatic infection, with a mean duration of infectivity longer than that of gonorrhea but substantially shorter than most HPV or genital HSV infections. Accordingly, chlamydia is more widespread in the population than gonorrhea but less so than HPV or herpes. Each of these STDs spreads within sexual networks, but the networks differ substantially from one another. Gonorrhea networks are largely limited to traditional core transmitters plus their occasional noncore sex partners, whereas genital herpes and HPV networks are extended, diverse, and long lasting.

The behavioral epidemiology of HIV/AIDS is unique among the STDs. HIV is transmissible for the life of an infected person, but infectivity is highly variable over that time—high soon after acquisition, low most of the time thereafter but punctuated by intervals of enhanced transmissibility, and higher again as immunodeficiency progresses. HIV transmission pressure is also influenced by circumcision status of men, occurrence of other inflammatory STDs, and access to therapy that can reduce viral load and transmission risk. Owing to these complex interactions, in most populations in industrialized countries HIV spreads like bacterial STDs, concentrated in core groups with high rates of concurrent partnerships or frequent partner change. By contrast, in many low-income countries HIV initially spreads rapidly in particularly high-risk individuals and later, as the epidemic matures, spreads more like herpes or HPV, producing generalized epidemics that place virtually the entire population at risk.

Sexual network theory helps explain why individual risk behaviors like number of partners or consistency of condom use may be poor predictors of STD infection, and why counseling individuals based on such risks may have modest influence on subsequent acquisition of HIV or other STDs. In generalized epidemics of HPV, HSV, or HIV infection, many persons whose own behavior implies low risk nonetheless become infected. A person may be monogamous, but his or her partner may have other partners, connecting the individual seemingly at low risk to a large sexual network. Within such networks, an important measure of epidemic potential is the frequency of concurrent partnerships, i.e. the formation of new partnerships are formed before preceding ones end. HIV/AIDS has become generalized in sub-Saharan Africa partly as a result of sex partner networks characterized by high rates of concurrency, even though the average number of sex partners is not substantially different than in the United States and most Western European countries where HIV/AIDS remains concentrated in selected population groups.

Differences in sexual networks also explain the often variable epidemiology of HIV/AIDS or other STDs among contiguous population groups. The incidence and prevalence of heterosexually transmitted HIV infection are as high in minority populations in Washington, DC, as in many sub-Saharan African countries, yet heterosexually transmitted HIV remains uncommon in most of the same city and its suburbs. Rates of most STDs are substantially higher in some racial/ethnic groups in the United States, notably African Americans, than in other groups, despite similar numbers of sex partners. These differences are largely explained by variations in concurrency rates and other aspects of sexual networks, rather than by numbers of sex partners or other measures that define core groups.

SEXUAL ORIENTATION

In the United States and most industrialized countries, men who have sex with men (MSM)—gay and bisexual men, plus others who may not acknowledge homosexual or bisexual orientation—had extraordinarily high rates of STDs in the 1970s and early 1980s, during which time HIV also was spreading rapidly, although largely unrecognized at the time. Rates of STDs and HIV infection in MSM then declined as a result of behavioral changes in response to AIDS, although the rates in MSM probably remained higher than those in most exclusively heterosexual populations. Similar trends occurred among MSM in most industrialized countries.

Since the late 1990s, the rates of STDs, and of HIV infections in some communities, have accelerated once more among MSM in the United States and other countries, a consequence of behavioral disinhibition, i.e., resurgent unsafe sexual behaviors following advances in HIV/AIDS treatment and survival. In the 2000s, accelerating rates in MSM have been documented for syphilis, gonorrhea and, where they have been studied, enteric infections and chlamydial infections, including lymphogranuloma venereum (LGV). The past decade has also seen increasing understanding of the high rate of anal cancer among MSM, the result of sexually transmitted HPV infection and perhaps accelerated progression to cancer among HIV infected persons. The greatest rises in reported STDs in the past decade, especially syphilis and LGV, have occurred among MSM already infected with HIV, perhaps in part because of "serosorting"—the practice of selecting partners with like HIV status. Clinicians who provide care to MSM, both with and without HIV infection, should not assume that their patients routinely follow safer sex guidelines; periodic STD screening and counseling are indicated for many such persons.

In contrast with MSM and exclusively heterosexual women and men, women who have sex with women (WSW) have relatively low rates of bacterial STDs like chlamydial infection, gonorrhea, and syphilis, but genital HPV infection and genital herpes seem to occur at rates similar to those in other population groups. Bacterial vaginosis (BV) is clearly and consistently transmitted sexually between women through shared vaginal secretions, and almost all female sex partners of WSW with BV are infected themselves. Clinicians should be alert to the possibility of STDs in WSW, including those who are exclusively lesbian.

INTERACTIONS BETWEEN HIV INFECTION AND OTHER STDs

Human immunodeficiency virus infection is the most devastating STD of all time, with mortality, morbidity, and social impact far exceeding those of syphilis in the pre–antibiotic era. Moreover, HIV interacts biologically with other STDs, and behavioral and social factors further contribute to the transmission of HIV. Most important, inflammatory STDs enhance the efficiency with which HIV is transmitted or acquired during sexual exposure. Genital herpes, syphilis, chancroid, gonorrhea, chlamydial infection, and trichomoniasis all have been shown in both cross-sectional and cohort studies to increase the likelihood of HIV transmission or acquisition by 2-fold to as much as 32-fold. In HIV-infected persons, many of the inflammatory cells recruited to infected mucosal surfaces or ulcers, such as macrophages and activated lymphocytes, are producing HIV in large numbers. In those without HIV infection, the same cells are especially susceptible to the virus if exposed.

Therefore, the prevalence of traditional STDs in a population strongly predicts the likelihood and frequency of sexual transmission of HIV. Indeed, the background prevalence and incidence of STDs is one of the main explanations for differences in the frequency of heterosexually transmitted HIV around the world and among populations within countries. On a population level, HSV-2 infection is the most important STD in enhancing HIV acquisition and transmission, with as many as half of all sexually transmitted HIV infections being directly attributable to the presence of HSV-2 in either the HIV-infected or susceptible partner.

Unfortunately, large randomized controlled trials have failed to demonstrate that antiherpetic therapy of HSV-2-infected persons prevented HIV acquisition or transmission. Other trials of STD treatment to prevent HIV transmission have given mixed results, with most studies showing no obvious impact, generating an ongoing debate about the utility of devoting HIV prevention resources to STD management. Most such studies were undertaken in populations with mature, generalized HIV epidemics, whereas modeling research suggests the impact of STD prevention is maximal during accelerating stage of an HIV epidemic, when HIV incidence is highest and transmission is driven largely by traditional core groups. For the clinician, there is no question that at the individual patient level, recognizing and treating inflammatory STDs carries benefits likely reduce HIV risk, and that primary prevention of genital herpes and other STDs has the potential to help curtail HIV transmission.

STDs also may adversely affect the clinical course of HIV disease, and vice versa. For example, among HIV-infected persons with recurrent genital herpes, HSV reactivation is accompanied by a rise in plasma HIV viral load, perhaps adversely affecting the progression of immunodeficiency. Aggressive, prolonged, and debilitating HSV infections were among the first opportunistic infections identified among AIDS patients, and HIV-infected persons have an elevated incidence of infection with acyclovir-resistant HSV strains. HIV infection also brings elevated rates of antibiotic treatment failure for syphilis and chancroid, possibly higher risks of neurological and ocular complications of syphilis, probably more rapid progression of genital or anal HPV infection to cancer, and perhaps higher frequency and severity of pelvic inflammatory disease.

STD HISTORY AND PHYSICAL EXAMINATION

Assessment of STD risk requires an accurate social and sexual history, including appraisal of factors that influence sexuality, such as substance abuse. A forthright, sensitive approach without value judgment usually elicits accurate information and often takes only 2 or 3 minutes. The medical history also can be succinct yet complete. The Appendix summarizes the sexual and medical histories, physical examination, and diagnostic tests undertaken routinely in the author's STD clinic.

The physical examination also is straightforward. All skin surfaces that are normally exposed during a genital examination are inspected quickly, including the face, head, hands, lower arms, lower trunk, pubic area, buttocks, and thighs. The mouth and throat are examined, and the neck and inguinal areas are palpated for lymphadenopathy. In men, the genitals and the pubic and inguinal regions are carefully inspected; the foreskin is retracted and inspected and the penis is palpated and "milked" to assess for urethral discharge; and the scrotal contents are palpated for masses, tenderness, and other abnormalities. For men who have had receptive anal intercourse, the anus and perineum are inspected. The examination of women includes meticulous inspection of the external genitals, perineum, and anus; speculum examination of the vagina and cervix; and a bimanual pelvic examination. For men or women with symptoms suggestive of proctitis or with lesions of the anus, the rectal mucosa is examined through an anoscope.

LABORATORY DIAGNOSIS

In industrialized countries, clinicians who manage patients with STD should have immediate access to serological tests for HIV infection and syphilis, including point-of-care rapid tests, as well as type-specific HSV antibody tests and nucleic acid amplification tests (NAAT) or culture for *Neisseria gonorrhoeae, C.*

trachomatis, and HSV. It is desirable to have immediate access to microscopy of Gram-stained or methylene blue-stained smears and wet mounts of vaginal secretions, although the Clinical Laboratory Improvement Act has made office-based microscopy problematical in some settings in the United States. Darkfield microscopy and rapid, point-of-care serological tests for syphilis ideally should be available.

- *Chlamydia trachomatis:* NAATs are the tests of choice. The currently available options are polymerase chain reaction (PCR) (e.g., Amplicor, Roche), transcription-mediated amplification (TMA) (e.g., Aptima, GenProbe), and the DNA strand displacement assay (SDA) (e.g., ProbeTec, BD Diagnostics).* Their sensitivities are 90–95%, compared with 70–80% for isolation in tissue culture and the older antigen-detection or nonamplified DNA probe tests. The NAATs retain excellent sensitivity on self-obtained vaginal swabs, recently certified by the U.S. Centers for Disease Control and Prevention (CDC) as the specimen of choice for *C. trachomatis* diagnosis and screening in women, and on urine in both men and women. Vaginal swab and urine specimens permit screening in settings where urethral or cervical sampling is impractical.

- *Neisseria gonorrhoeae:* All cases of gonorrhea should be confirmed by specific laboratory tests. Isolation of *N. gonorrhoeae* by culture has largely been supplanted by NAATs, using the same types as for identification of *C. trachomatis.** Combination tests for simultaneous identification of both organisms are the norm in many clinical settings. Unlike the chlamydia tests, however, culture of *N. gonorrhoeae* remains highly sensitive and inexpensive, and has the advantage of preserving isolates for antimicrobial susceptibility testing.

- Herpes simplex virus: Culture or NAAT to detect HSV is indicated for all sexually active patients with genital ulcer disease. Even when the diagnosis is apparent on clinical grounds, virologic methods are required to determine virus type, because the clinical course and management are significantly different between HSV-1 and HSV-2. PCR for HSV is increasingly available in the United States and most industrialized countries, is substantially more sensitive than virus isolation, and is the test of choice.

- HSV serology: Type-specific serological assays for immunoglobulin G (IgG) antibody to HSV, which accurately distinguish herpes simplex virus type 2 (HSV-2) from HSV type 1 (HSV-1) antibody, are indicated as a diagnostic aid in patients with genital ulcer disease, to evaluate the partners of persons with genital herpes, and (somewhat controversially) for screening in selected populations. Although immunoglobulin M (IgM) serological tests for HSV are offered by some laboratories, they have little or no role in clinical management. Contrary to some infections, IgM antibody often does not precede IgG antibody in initial HSV infections and often persists in chronic herpes, so that testing does not reliably differentiate early from longstanding infection. Further, false-positive results are common in patients without HSV infection and no type-specific HSV IgM assays are available. Clinicians are encouraged to not request HSV IgM antibody tests, and to disregard either positive or negative results if laboratories perform IgM testing without request.

---

* At the time of writing, evidence suggests that the main commercially available PCR and SDA tests for *N. gonorrhoeae,* and PCR for *C. trachomatis,* have lower specificities than TMA, resulting in an unacceptably high rate of false-positive results in low prevalence settings. PCR, therefore, should be used with caution, if at all, in populations with low prevalences of either infection. However, all NAATs are subject to modification by the manufacturer or, in some cases, by modified test procedures by individual laboratories, and improved performance may be expected in some settings.

- HIV serology: Tests for antibody to HIV should be done routinely in all persons with STD or at risk. Combination tests that detect both antibody to HIV and the HIV p24 surface antigen improve sensitivity in early infection (≤4 weeks) and are especially useful in screening populations at high risk, such as MSM, injection drug users, and persons recently exposed to infected partners. Both laboratory-based and rapid, point-of-care antibody tests are available. Positive results for all antibody tests require confirmation by Western blot or other confirmatory test. Positive results on two separate antibody tests also offer acceptable evidence of infection without reliance on Western blot confirmation, a useful strategy in resource-poor settings. NAAT to detect HIV RNA in serum can further shorten the diagnostic window period and is indicated when there is clinical suspicion of primary HIV infection or, by testing pooled sera, to detect acute HIV infection in selected high-prevalence settings.

- Serological tests for syphilis: Antibody tests for syphilis are indicated for screening of most or all patients being evaluated for STD. The historical standard is to test initially with nontreponemal antibody tests, such as the Venereal Disease Research Laboratory (VDRL), rapid plasma reagin (RPR), or toluidine red unheated serum reagin test (TRUST), and to confirm positive results by various *Treponema pallidum*-specific antibody tests, such as the *T. pallidum* particle agglutination (TPPA) or fluorescent treponemal antibody-absorbed (FTA-ABS) test. However, with the development of inexpensive, readily automated enzyme immunoassays (EIAs) and other tests for *T. pallidum*-specific antibody, the historical standard has been reversed in many settings. EIA and similar assays, including *T. pallidum*-specific point-of-care tests, are increasingly employed for initial testing followed by a quantitative RPR or VDRL test to assess disease activity.

- Viral hepatitis serology: Serological tests for past or current viral hepatitis (A, B, or C) are useful in some populations and should be readily available in STD clinical settings.

- Vaginal pathogens: The most common causes of vaginal discharge in young women, bacterial vaginosis (BV), trichomoniasis, vulvovaginal candidiasis, and mucopurulent cervicitis, often are difficult to differentiate clinically, and require microscopy or microbiologic tests. Rapid, point-of-care tests for semiquantitation of *Gardnerella vaginalis* or other rapid test methods are available for the diagnosis of BV and may supplant microscopic examination in some settings. NAAT is becoming the diagnostic standard for *Trichomonas vaginalis*; it has double the sensitivity of microscopy for detection in women and is the only test that reliably detects *T. vaginalis* in men.

- Cervical or anal cancer screening and HPV: Papanicolaou smears should be available in clinical settings that serve patients with STD. The age at which women should be routinely tested and the recommended frequency of screening are in evolution; clinicians should monitor local and regional recommendations. NAAT for HPV increasingly accompanies cervical cytology, and is an important tool for prevention of cervical cancer in developing countries where cervical cytology is impractical. The role of routine HPV testing in industrialized countries, independent of cervical cytology, is uncertain and controversial. Anal cytology has been advocated as a screening test in MSM who have had receptive anal intercourse, but is not presently recommended routinely.

- Other pathogens: NAATs for *Mycoplasma genitalium* and *Ureaplasma urealyticum* are increasingly available. Routine diagnostic testing or screening for these organisms is not currently recommended, but testing may have proved useful in evaluation of men with nongonococcal urethritis (NGU), especially when NGU persists or recurs after treatment. Assays for newly described bacterial vaginosis-associated bacteria (BVAB types 1, 2, and 3) may become commercially available, but their clinical utility is unknown.

SCREENING AND THE ROUTINE STD EVALUATION

Screening for STD Screening means laboratory testing for STDs in persons at risk, in the absence of symptoms, other clinical evidence of infection, or known STD exposure. When practical, persons at high risk should be screened whenever they present for health care for any reason. With modern tests and specimen collection methods, STD screening generally can be accomplished with minimal impact on care for the problem that brings a patient to the office or clinic. The STDs for which screening is indicated depends on patient characteristics such as age, sex, gender of partners, local prevalence of specific infections, test performance, the potential impact of case detection on patient's health, the frequency and costs of the sequelae that might be prevented by early detection, the direct cost of the test, and indirect costs, such as the convenience and time required for the test procedure. Screening has a central role in the control of chlamydial infection, gonorrhea, HIV, cervical cancer, and probably syphilis, and may be useful in selected settings to prevent genital or neonatal herpes.

Screening for HIV CDC recommends that in the United States, all persons aged 13–64 be tested once for HIV when they attend for routine health care (for any reason), using an opt-out approach that assumes testing unless the patient requests otherwise, and without written consent or required risk assessment or counseling. The recommendation is supported by data showing that many persons with HIV are unaware they are infected or, sometimes, that they are at risk; that knowingly infected persons are less likely to transmit HIV; that pre-test risk assessment and counseling have come to be viewed as barriers to testing; the high morbidity and costs associated with HIV infection, especially when diagnosed late; and the availability of highly accurate, low-cost tests. Opt-out testing in pregnant woman and all blood and organ donors is accepted nearly universally by patients and is responsible for the near eradication of HIV transmission perinatally and by transfusion and organ transplantation in the United States and most other industrialized countries. The same approach should be considered the standard of care in all health care settings. Routine HIV screening also is increasingly employed in developing countries, often in the form of provider-initiated testing and counseling (PITC).

Routine STD Evaluation Sometimes asymptomatic patients present with requests for comprehensive STD assessment. The patient's age and other factors will determine the specific tests. Because chlamydial infection is common in all settings and populations, a test for *C. trachomatis* generally should be done in both men and heterosexual women, especially in persons ≤25 years old. The need for gonorrhea testing depends on the local prevalence of infection and the patient's risk history, but most patients tested for either chlamydia or gonorrhea typically are tested for both, because NAATs for *C. trachomatis* and *N. gonorrhoeae* often are linked at little or no increased cost.

Most patients who request evaluation for STD will expect and should have HIV testing. Routine screening for HSV infection is controversial, but with the ready availability of type-specific HSV serological tests, patients requesting comprehensive STD screening should be informed of the option to have a type-specific HSV-2 antibody test. Women should be evaluated for the common vulvovaginal infections, which may be asymptomatic. Both men and women should be examined for anogenital warts, ulcers, and other lesions. The need for a serological test for syphilis in many heterosexual patients has declined, as the incidence of syphilis has fallen to very low levels in most populations in the United States. However, testing is inexpensive and many patients expect routine syphilis screening.

Screening for hepatitis B is of uncertain value for most heterosexual patients in the United States and other industrialized countries, if there are no risks for exposure to infected blood, such as injection drug use. (Routine immunization, without screening, is recommended.) Contrary to popular perceptions, hepatitis C is rarely sexually transmitted; screening is indicated in persons at risk for blood exposure, such as injection drug users, who commonly present for STD services—but not generally on the basis of STD risk per se. In industrialized countries, screening NAAT for HPV generally recommended primarily as supplemental analysis of cervical Pap smears, but HPV screening tests per se may have an important role in cervical cancer prevention in developing countries.

MSM who request STD evaluation generally should be tested for urethral gonorrhea and chlamydial infection, for rectal infection if they participate in anal receptive intercourse, and for pharyngeal gonococcal infection. Pharyngeal chlamydial infection is too rare to warrant routine screening, even if a validated or approved assay is available. HIV testing and syphilis testing should be routine, and screening for HSV-2 is recommended by some experts, owing to the high prevalence of infection and its contribution to the risk of HIV infection. Hepatitis B and hepatitis A antibody testing may be warranted, depending on past infection or immunization history. Anal cytology is recommended by some experts but is not routine in most settings.

Formal STD screening guidelines are lacking for WSW, but those who have sex with both female and male partners should be screened in the same manner as women who exclusively have sex with men. Women who have sex only with women should be screened for vaginal infections and HIV and should undergo cervical cytology (with or without HPV testing) according to standard guidelines. Testing for bacterial STDs is likely to have a low yield but should be done if the sex of the patient's partners is not known with certainty.

Screening Frequency Few guidelines address STD screening frequency. For sexually active young adults (≤25 years old) outside mutually monogamous relationships, annual screening for common STDs and HIV probably is reasonable. For women, this often can be accomplished during routine reproductive health visits. Sexually active teens should be tested for *C. trachomatis* at least annually and whenever they attend for routine health care, regardless of frequency. Sexually active persons at particularly high risk for HIV, such as MSM, injection drug users, and commercial sex workers should be tested regularly at intervals that may range from 3 to 12 months, depending on frequency of sexual encounters or other risk factors.

PRINCIPLES OF STD TREATMENT

Etiologic treatment, i.e., therapy directed toward a documented pathogen, is often considered the ideal approach, but most patients with STDs are treated presumptively, before diagnostic test results are available. Most chlamydial infections in men are treated when they present with nongonococcal urethritis (NGU). Similarly, many patients with gonorrhea, syphilis, genital herpes, and other STDs, and their sex partners, are treated presumptively while awaiting test results, in order to maximize therapeutic effectiveness, prevent complications, and prevent transmission. True etiologic treatment is most commonly employed when screening detects infection in the absence of symptoms or signs.

Syndromic management is diagnosis and therapy on the basis of standardized clinical and epidemiologic criteria, usually with no attempt at etiologic diagnosis. A necessary strategy in many resource-poor settings, syndromic management has been credited with significant reductions in STD rates in some settings in developing countries. However, syndromic management is inherently limited in its ability to control STDs at the population level owing to high frequencies of asymptomatic infection for most STDs. Syndromic management has a limited role in STD management in industrialized countries, and its utility in developing countries should be viewed as a necessary stopgap until the day when low-cost NAATs and serological tests for common STDs become readily available. A further limitation of syndromic management is uncertainty about what treatment(s), if any, to administer to patients' sex partners. The STD syndromic management recommendations of the World Health Organization are summarized in Chap. 2.

Several STDs respond well to single-dose treatment, obviating the risks of treatment failure and continued transmission that can result from poor compliance with multiple-dose regimens. Directly observed single-dose treatment has a special role in STD management and is the preferred mode for chlamydial infection, gonorrhea, chancroid, trichomoniasis, and syphilis. Directly observed treatment for STDs preceded the reliance on this approach as a mainstay of tuberculosis management by several decades.

MANAGEMENT OF SEX PARTNERS

Management of patients' sex partners is integral to STD clinical care. With few exceptions, the partners of persons with bacterial STDs should be treated presumptively, without awaiting the results of specific diagnostic tests. Testing nonetheless should be routine, because both patients' and their partners' understanding of the importance of compliance, follow-up, and successful treatment of any additional sex partners are largely contingent on documented infection. Failure to assure treatment of the partner often is tantamount to not treating the index patient, who may be reinfected, and fosters spread to additional persons. In some geographic areas of the United States and in some other countries, local, state or provincial health agencies may assist in partner notification and management for syphilis or HIV infection, but centralized partner services rarely are available for gonorrhea, chlamydial infection, or other STDs. Accordingly, the clinician must advise his or her patients to inform their partners and assist in assuring treatment. Euphemisms and obfuscation about the nature of the clinical condition should be avoided; partners should understand what STD was diagnosed and why treatment is necessary.

When practical, partners should be examined in person, tested, treated, and counseled. This was historically the only approach recommended by CDC and other prevention agencies for STD partner management. However, it has long been apparent that many partners fail to seek medical care, resulting in reinfection of index patients and sustained transmission in the community. In response, clinicians often arranged for treatment of partners without examination, typically by providing extra drug to the index patient or by writing a prescription for the partner. This strategy is now called expedited partner therapy (EPT) or patient-delivered partner therapy (PDPT). EPT has historically been routinely employed for the male partners of women with vaginal trichomoniasis.

Several randomized controlled trials have now shown EPT to be effective for chlamydial infection and gonorrhea and substantially superior to traditional partner management, with higher rates of documented treatment, reduced frequency of repeat sex with untreated partners, and, most important, reduced frequency of recurrent infection among index patients. CDC now recommends EPT as a routine option to ensure treatment of the partners of heterosexual men and women with chlamydial infection or gonorrhea. Insufficient data are available to support routine use of EPT among MSM, in whom a high proportion might have other undiagnosed STDs, especially HIV infection. Nevertheless, EPT should be considered in MSM when necessary to ensure treatment of partners. Somewhat surprisingly, there are conflicting data on the value of EPT for trichomoniasis, but the strategy nevertheless makes sense in some settings, perhaps especially when other STDs are not likely to be present simultaneously. No data are available on the utility or necessity of EPT in the management of nonchlamydial NGU or mucopurulent cervicitis, and EPT is not practical for syphilis, which requires penicillin by injection, or for viral STDs.

PREVENTION COUNSELING

Condoms, Abstinence, and Monogamy Clinicians who manage persons with STD should help their patients reduce the risk of infection in the future. Sexual safety should be addressed with all young people, with the same forthright but sensitive approach used for medical and sexual histories. Regardless of the clinician's personal views on community standards or other aspects of sexual behavior, he or she should understand that most persons at risk will more readily accept education and counseling based on pragmatic rationales than on moral or religious grounds. Sexual abstinence or limitation of sexual activity to a single partner in a mutually monogamous relationship should be described for appropriate patients as the surest approaches to STD prevention. However, these options present insurmountable barriers for most patients, and abstinence and monogamy should never be the sole prevention advice. Consistent use of condoms should be strongly recommended for nonmonogamous vaginal or anal intercourse, but condoms and other barriers may be considered optional for oral sex, which carries lower risks of STD transmission. Owing to extremely high rates of STD in sexually active teenagers, related to both concurrency and rapid partner changes ("serial monogamy"), most unmarried persons <20 years old should be encouraged to use condoms for all vaginal or anal sexual exposures, even in committed relationships.

Partner Selection and Concurrency Counseling should address selectivity in choosing sexual partners, the recognition and response to symptoms of STD, and the links between STD and substance abuse and between HIV infection and other STDs. The importance of avoiding simultaneous partnerships has been increasingly recognized through improved understanding of sexual networks. Patients can be counseled that unprotected sex with new partners should be deferred until prior relationships have ended. It also is worthwhile to advise patients to avoid situations and settings that are especially conducive to high-risk sexual behavior, such as alcohol ingestion, use of recreational drugs, and places where anonymous sexual encounters are expected.

CASE REPORTING

Data on STD morbidity and local and regional epidemiology are essential for the rational design of prevention programs and to leverage resources for public health intervention. Further, these resources can be directed to populations and communities at risk only if their occurrence, location, and demographic characteristics are known. Chlamydial infection, gonorrhea, syphilis, hepatitis B, and AIDS are universally reportable in most industrialized countries, and HIV infection in the absence of overt AIDS increasingly so. In addition to collating statistics and undertaking epidemiologic analysis, health departments often use case reports of syphilis or HIV infection to initiate confidential partner notification. Clinicians should be familiar with local regulations and report all cases of designated STDs.

SUGGESTED READING

Barnabas RV, Wasserheit JN. Riddle of the Sphinx revisited: the role of STDs in HIV prevention. *Sex Transm Dis.* 2009;36:365-7. *A succinct review of the trials of STD management for STD prevention, including the importance of core groups and sexual networks in STD/HIV transmission.*

Branson BM, et al. Centers for Disease Control and Prevention. Revised recommendations for HIV testing of adults, adolescents, and pregnant women in health-care settings. *MMWR.* 2006;55(RR-14):1-17. http://www.cdc.gov/mmwr/preview/mmwrhtml/rr5514a1.htm. Accessed January 14, 2011. *CDC policy statement and recommendations for routine opt-out HIV testing as the central strategy to prevent HIV/AIDS in the United States.*

Centers for Disease Control and Prevention. Recommendations for partner services programs for HIV infection, syphilis, gonorrhea and chlamydial infection. *MMWR.* 2008;57(RR-9):1-85. http://www.cdc.gov/nchhstp/partners/Recommendations.html. Accessed January 14, 2011. *Evidence based approaches to assure partner notification, diagnosis and treatment.*

Centers for Disease Control and Prevention. Sexually transmitted diseases treatment guidelines, 2010. MMWR 2010; 59:RR-12:1-110. http://www.cdc.gov/std/treatment/2010/default.htm. Accessed January 14, 2011. *CDC's evidence based recommendations for diagnosis and management of STDs.*

Handsfield HH, et al. Expedited partner therapy in the management of sexually transmitted infections. Centers for Disease Control and Prevention., 2006:1-53. http://www.cdc.gov/std/treatment/EPTFinal-Report2006.pdf. Accessed January 14, 2011. *A comprehensive review of the data that support of CDC's recommendations for routine use of EPT for chlamydial infection and gonorrhea.*

Holmes KK, et al, eds. *Sexually Transmitted Diseases.* 4th ed. New York, NY: McGraw-Hill;2008 (2,166 pp). *The definitive textbook on STDs.*

Morris M, et al. Concurrent partnerships and HIV prevalence disparities by race: linking science and public health practice. *Am J Public Health.* 2009;99:1023-31. *A study explaining the importance of concurrency as an influence on STD/HIV transmission and a useful introduction to the concept of sex partner networks.*

The Medical Letter on Drugs and Therapeutics. Drugs for sexually transmitted infections. Treatment guidelines from The Medical Letter 2010:8(95). *A succinct review of STD treatment options, with recommendations similar to the CDC guidelines.*

2

Global Epidemiology, Prevention and Management of Sexually Transmitted Diseases

Judd L. Walson, Laura Sangaré, and H. Hunter Handsfield

EPIDEMIOLOGY AND PREVENTION

Sexually transmitted diseases (STDs) are a major cause of morbidity and mortality throughout the world, with significant public health impact. Differences in populations at risk, methods of detection, and strategies for management all result in significant geographic variation in the epidemiology and optimal prevention strategies. While encouraging trends have been noted in the decreasing incidence of some conditions, such as chancroid and syphilis, viral STDs such as infection with herpes simplex virus type 2 (HSV-2) and the human immunodeficiency viruses (HIV) are rising in incidence and prevalence, particularly in developing countries, where prevention and control are high priorities on the global health agenda.

The World Health Organization (WHO) estimates that >90% of the global STD burden occurs in developing countries (see Table 2–1). HIV-1, and secondarily HIV-2, have had a devastating impact, particularly in sub-Saharan Africa, where two-thirds of all people living with HIV reside and two-thirds of all new HIV infections occur each year. Of the more than 340 million annual new cases of curable STDs (chlamydia, gonorrhea, syphilis, and trichomoniasis) in adults aged 15 to 49 years, the highest incidence rates occur in south and southeast Asia (about 151 million infections per year) and sub-Saharan Africa (69 million per year). In addition, southern Africa has the highest prevalence of existing STDs, with an estimated 119 infections per 1,000 members of the population, followed by Latin America and the Caribbean, which together are estimated to have about 71 STDs per 1,000 people, and all these rates continue to rise steadily. The consequences are enormous, owing both to their direct health consequences and their impact on the economic growth and productivity of populations. The HIV epidemic

Table 2–1 ESTIMATED ANNUAL INCIDENCE OF CURABLE SEXUALLY TRANSMITTED DISEASES GLOBALLY, 1999*

Region	No. of New Infections per Year
South and Southeast Asia	151 million
Sub-Saharan Africa	69 million
Latin America and the Caribbean	38 million
Eastern Europe and Central Asia	22 million
East Asia and the Pacific	18 million
Western Europe	17 million
North America	14 million
North Africa and the Middle East	10 million
Australia and New Zealand	1 million
Total	340 million

Data from World Health Organization. Available at http://www.who.int/hiv/pub/sti/who_hiv_aids_2001.02.pdf (accessed September 24, 2010). Curable STDs include chlamydial infection, gonorrhea, syphilis, and trichomoniasis. Updated estimates from WHO are anticipated in the near future.

alone is one of the major constraints on the social and economic progress of countries like South Africa, Zimbabwe, Botswana, Uganda, Jamaica, and Trinidad & Tobago, among several others.

Table 2–2 lists some of the main public health impacts of HIV and other STDs. HIV/AIDS ranks as a leading cause of death in many countries, especially in persons under 40 years of age. Beyond mortality per se, a common measure of such impact is *disability-adjusted life years* (DALYs), which takes into account both early death and the effects of impaired functioning, lost productivity, and time spent in

Table 2–2 ESTIMATED GLOBAL MORTALITY AND DISABILITY IMPACT OF HIV/AIDS, SYPHILIS, CHLAMYDIAL INFECTION, AND GONORRHEA, 2004*

	Female		Male		Total	
	Deaths	DALYs[†]	Deaths	DALYs[†]	Deaths	DALYs[†]
HIV/AIDS	1.01 million	29.9 million	1.03 million	28.6 million	2.04 million	58.5 million
Syphilis	39,000	1.3 million	60,000	1.5 million	99,000	2.8 million
Chlamydia	9,000	3.4 million	—	320,000	9,000	3.7 million
Gonorrhea	500	2.0 million	500	1.6 million	1,000	3.6 million

*Adapted from data compiled by the World Health Organization.
[†]DALYs = disability-adjusted life years and computes the functional impact of health problems by estimating the number of healthy years of life lost due to the combined effects of disability and premature death.

health care. Substantial disease burden results from ulcerative and inflammatory STDs owing largely to their contribution to acquisition and transmission of HIV.

As discussed in Chap. 1, STDs are sexist in their impact; while all individuals with STD suffer directly or indirectly, women and their children are disproportionately affected. STDs are the leading preventable causes of infertility in developing countries and probably in industrialized countries as well, and result in millions of cases of pelvic inflammatory disease (PID) and life-threatening ectopic pregnancy. An estimated 25% of all miscarriages and stillbirths worldwide are attributed to syphilis. Perinatally transmitted HIV has caused millions of early deaths among young children, and HIV infection in parents has orphaned many more. Beyond these fatal impacts on newborns and young children, STDs also are a common cause globally of low birth weight, blindness, neurodevelopmental delay, and pneumonia.

Virtually by definition, STDs disproportionately affect the most sexually active men and women, which in most of the world predominantly are those between ages 15 and 35 years. Accordingly, part of the rising impact of STDs is fueled by demographic trends. For example, in most developing countries, the proportion of the population in the maximally sexually active years is substantially greater than in most industrialized nations, helping propel high rates of HIV/AIDS and other STDs. While some factors, such as living in urban areas with high unemployment and engaging in sex work, confer greater risk of STD acquisition, many sexual behavior patterns are different across regions and countries. Populations at high risk include the world's increasingly mobile populations, especially refugees and displaced persons, military personnel, orphaned or abused children and adolescents, and women forced into the sex trade. These and other demographic, social, and infrastructural determinants of STD rates operate largely by their influence on partner selection, concurrency, sex partner network structure, and often access to health care (see Chap. 1).

Effective prevention and control of STDs requires strategies that address both populations and individuals. By itself, no particular prevention strategy, even strong biomedical ones like condom promotion, male circumcision, and increased case finding through testing, is likely to substantially curtail the spread of HIV and other STDs. Successful prevention must be based on combinations of methods, integrating biomedical approaches with promotion of healthy sexual behavior, provision of barrier protection, improved access to care for STDs and HIV treatment, and effective data gathering and surveillance. These multifaceted strategies must be implemented throughout society, to include not only clinical facilities but schools, government agencies, nongovernmental organizations, community groups, religious institutions, and families. Also largely missing in many countries most affected by AIDS and STDs is strong advocacy from governments, funding agencies, and other leaders to mobilize the programmatic and political commitments to respond effectively to the threat of STDs.

DIAGNOSIS AND MANAGEMENT OF STDs

Prevention and control of STDs requires accurate diagnosis of infected individuals and effective therapy for treatable infections and complications. Laboratory screening to detect subclinical infections also is desirable and often necessary for successful prevention. In most industrialized countries, diagnostic testing for STDs is routinely performed in symptomatic individuals, screening tests of asymptomatic persons may be offered among selected populations, and case detection through diagnosis and screening in turn allow specific anti-infective therapy. However, most developing countries lack the resources to permit laboratory-based screening or diagnostic testing. Inadequate laboratory infrastructure, difficult supply chain management, insufficient numbers of trained personnel, and high expense are major barriers, problems often compounded by limited availability of the most effective treatments.

Syndromic management of STDs evolved in response to the lack of available diagnostic testing in resource-limited settings. First developed and implemented in Zimbabwe and other southern African countries, syndromic management has been incorporated into guidelines promoted by WHO and others for use when etiologic diagnosis is not readily available. Syndromic management relies on the clinical identification of standard groups of easily recognized signs and symptoms (syndromes) and provides easy-to-follow algorithms for the management and treatment of common STDs, without reliance on laboratory-confirmed diagnosis. Syndromic management for urethral discharge in men (Fig. 2–1) has proved to be feasible, effective, and cost-effective in resource-limited settings for treating gonorrhea and chlamydial infection. (However, the rapid evolution and spread of fluoroquinolone-resistant *Neisseria gonorrhoeae* has become a difficult challenge in many settings; see Chap. 3.)

Syndromic management of genital ulcer disease (GUD) in men and women, designed primarily to ensure proper treatment of syphilis and chancroid (Fig. 2–2), also has proved effective and feasible and may be credited in part for the declining frequency of chancroid and perhaps syphilis in some countries.

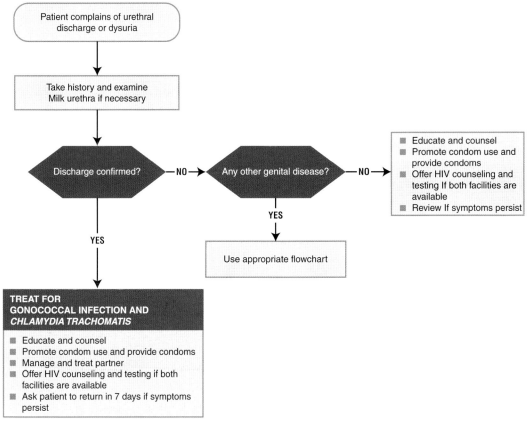

2–1. World Health Organization recommended syndromic management of men with urethral discharge. (*World Health Organization. Guidelines for the management of sexually transmitted infections. Geneva, WHO, 2003. Fig 1. http://www.who.int/hiv/pub/sti/pub6/en/STIGuidelines2003.pdf. Accessed February 1, 2011.*)

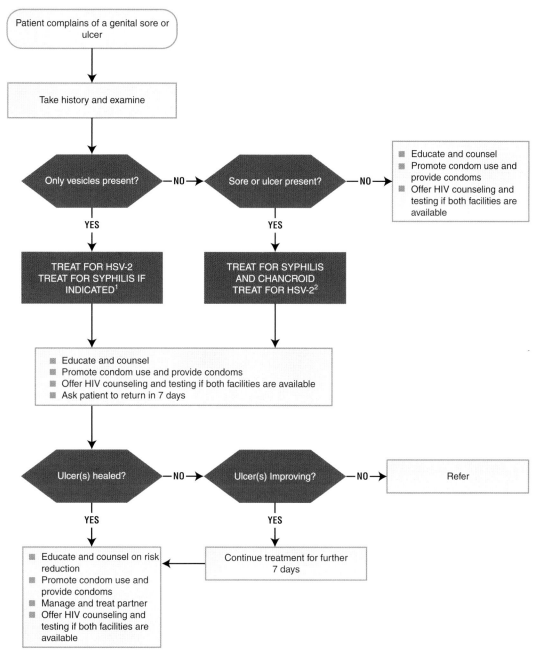

2–2. World Health Organization recommended syndromic management of patients with genital ulcer disease. (*World Health Organization. Guidelines for the management of sexually transmitted infections. Geneva, WHO, 2003. Fig 3. http://www.who.int/hiv/pub/sti/pub6/en/STIGuidelines2003.pdf. Accessed February 1, 2011.*)

At the same time, however, the contribution of genital herpes to GUD has risen dramatically in many developing countries, creating a virulent, bidirectional epidemiologic synergy that fuels, and is fueled by, rising rates of HIV/AIDS (see Chap. 8). Rising herpes and declining chancroid and perhaps syphilis now challenge the effectiveness of the current syndromic management recommendations for GUD. In response, by 2010 a few countries (e.g., Botswana) had changed their GUD protocols, and modified GUD syndromic management guidelines by WHO are anticipated.

In contrast to the relative success of syndromic management of GUD and urethral discharge in men, syndromic management of vaginal discharge, intended largely as a surrogate for cervicitis to ensure effective treatment of gonorrhea and chlamydia, has been less successful. This reflects the multiple potential etiologies of vaginal discharge and resulting low specificity of discharge and other vulvovaginal symptoms as makers of STD in general and of gonorrhea and chlamydia in particular.

Although syndromic management of STDs may have contributed to reduced rates of gonorrhea, chancroid, and perhaps syphilis in some settings, and is credited with helping reduce the incidence of HIV infection in one randomized controlled trial in Tanzania, there are serious limitations to syndromic management. As noted, syndromic management of vaginal discharge has had no demonstrable benefit in controlling gonorrhea or chlamydial infection. Even if improved guidelines allow better recognition of HSV-2 infections, effective treatment of herpes is a challenge in many resource-limited settings. Further, effective syndromic management requires reassessment of possible fluctuations in the etiologies of the syndromes and their optimal treatment, by periodic or ongoing surveillance of current etiologic diagnoses and antimicrobial susceptibility. Almost by definition, the means and infrastructure for such revalidation of syndromic guidelines are lacking in those places most reliant on them. Thus, the replacement of chancroid with herpes among patients with GUD went undetected for a decade or more in some countries, and treatment of gonorrhea with fluoroquinolones remains common in many settings where resistance probably is prevalent.

Perhaps most important, the effectiveness of syndromic management for STD control will always be limited by its reliance on symptoms that bring patients to clinical facilities. Both subclinical infection and lack of easy access to clinical services guarantee that at best a minority of infected persons can be reached. Further, successful partner management largely depends on etiologic diagnosis. It is challenging enough to advise asymptomatic partners to seek clinical care, and undoubtedly more so when the index case cannot be given a specific diagnosis. It is also more difficult to employ strategies like expedited partner therapy without an etiologic diagnosis. Rapid, inexpensive, low technology diagnostic tests are increasingly available for HIV infection and syphilis, and promising research is under way for such tests for *Chlamydia trachomatis*, *N. gonorrhoeae*, *Trichomonas vaginalis*, *Haemophilis ducreyi*, and HSV-2. But until they are readily available at low cost, syndromic management will remain the standard of STD clinical care in many settings.

INTERNATIONAL ASPECTS OF SELECTED STDs

HIV Infection and AIDS

Epidemiology HIV/AIDS is the most serious and important STD of all time and its prevention is a priority in WHO's Millennium Development Goals. Over 33 million individuals worldwide are living with HIV infection, more than 2.7 million new infections are estimated to occur annually, and annual mortality exceeds 2 million people. The news is not all bleak, however. Antiretroviral therapy (ART) is becoming more available even in some of the world's poorest countries, and in recent years some progress has been made in reducing incident infections. With improved prevention, the number of new infections is believed to have declined by approximately one-third from the mid-1990s through 2010. Nevertheless, it has been estimated that in 2010, there were 5 new HIV infections for every two persons who began ART.

As for all STDs, the epidemiology of HIV is notable for major geographical differences in prevalence and incidence. Two-thirds of all people with HIV and 70% of all new infections occur in sub-Saharan Africa, where overall adult prevalence exceeds 20% in some countries. HIV prevalence is lower in Asia than Africa, but because of its enormous population, Asia has only modestly fewer newly HIV-infected persons than Africa. Fewer than 5% of HIV-infected persons reside in eastern Europe, but this region is particularly important in the global epidemiology of HIV because of great population migration out of the region, contributing to international spread. Despite the relatively small population in the Caribbean, that region has some of the most impacted countries and suffers the highest prevalence of HIV other than southern Africa.

In addition to differences in prevalence and incidence, there is significant geographic variability in the predominant modes of transmission and the population groups at highest risk. In southern Africa, the Caribbean, and parts of India and China, most incident HIV infections result from heterosexual transmission, whereas sex between men is the dominant mode of transmission in Latin America, North America, and western Europe. The combination of injection drug use (with shared injection equipment) and heterosexual transmission, often through commercial sex, has been particularly important in eastern Europe. In many parts of Asia, sex workers and their clients, injection drug users, and men who have sex with men (MSM) have been traditional high-risk groups, accounting for a large proportion of new infections. Mother-to-child transmission of HIV has been almost completely eliminated in many countries, especially in North America and western Europe, but both perinatal transmission and postnatal transmission through breastfeeding remain important modes of infection in Africa and some other regions.

As a consequence of these highly variable transmission dynamics and populations at risk, at the country-level HIV epidemics have been characterized as *low-level*, *concentrated*, and *generalized*. In low-level epidemics, HIV infection may have existed for many years but has not yet spread to significant levels in any subpopulation, and there is no defined population group in which HIV prevalence exceeds 5%. Recorded infections are generally limited to scattered individuals with particularly high-risk behaviors, such as sex workers, injection drug users, and MSM, and transmission networks tend to be diffuse. Japan, the Philippines, China, and most countries of northern Africa and the Middle East are examples of countries with low-level epidemics (as of the late 2000s). In concentrated HIV epidemics, HIV has spread rapidly in one or more defined subpopulations. In those groups, >5% of individuals are infected, but transmission is not yet well established in the general population. Transmission networks tend to be concentrated within high-risk subgroups and the prevalence of HIV infection in pregnant women is <1%. The United States, India, and most European and Latin American countries have concentrated epidemics. Finally, in generalized epidemics HIV is well established in the general population, sexual networks within the broad population sustain transmission, and among pregnant women 1% or more are infected. Most countries of sub-Saharan Africa and several Caribbean nations have generalized HIV epidemics.

Diagnosis The diagnosis of HIV infection is most often based on the detection of serum antibody to HIV antigens. Standard assays are based on enzyme immunoassay (EIA) screening with confirmatory testing of EIA-positive samples by Western blot. Currently available assays detect all subtypes of HIV with a high degree of accuracy. Positive EIA results are highly sensitive when performed sufficiently long after acquisition of HIV, and the combination of positive EIA and Western blot is virtually

100% specific. In many areas of the world, rapid, point-of-care antibody testing of blood or oral fluids, which does not require sophisticated laboratories, has become the standard method for HIV diagnosis. Although somewhat less sensitive and specific than standard EIA, these tests are inexpensive, require minimal training, and provide results within minutes, obviating difficulties in conveying results in places with challenges to communication and travel. In resource-limited settings, positive results on two rapid tests by separate manufacturers is equally specific as EIA confirmed by Western blot, and dual rapid testing is the diagnostic norm in many developing countries.

Serologic testing may fail to detect an antibody response during acute HIV infection, i.e., in the 2–6 weeks before seroconversion, and may detect maternal HIV antibody in infants under 18 months of age, resulting in false-positive diagnosis of HIV in the child. Combination assays for both HIV antibody and HIV p24 antigen partly address this issue, detecting nearly 100% of incident HIV infections as soon as 4 weeks after infection, and can be useful in evaluating persons at particularly high risk of new HIV infection. Nucleic acid amplification tests (NAATs) to detect HIV RNA also are available and still more sensitive in detecting early infection, usually becoming positive within 10 days of infection. However, combination antigen-antibody assays and NAATs remain expensive and technically demanding, making them unavailable for use in many areas most severely impacted by the HIV pandemic.

HIV Prevention Strategies The use of testing and counseling as strategies to control HIV evolved in important ways in the 2000s. Counseling uninfected persons often is followed by less frequent self-reported risky behaviors, but actual behavior change has been difficult to document and reduced rates of HIV infection have not been demonstrated. In contrast, persons found to be HIV infected have markedly reduced risk behaviors thereafter—probably spontaneously, but likely strengthened by counseling—making them substantially less likely to transmit the virus. As the HIV pandemic evolved over two decades, the easiest to reach infected persons were increasingly tested and diagnosed (the "low hanging fruit"), and the proportion of infected people who were unaware of their risks rose steadily. Therefore, risk-based testing became progressively less productive in identifying infected persons. Further, strategies initially considered facilitators of test acceptance—pre-test risk assessment and counseling, formal informed consent, in-person test results, and universal post-test counseling—came to be viewed as barriers instead. Pre-test risk assessment and counseling is viewed by many at risk as a requirement to reveal their deepest personal secrets as a condition of testing, whereas testing usually is readily accepted when presented as routine for all patients. Routine testing with opt-out consent was an important contributor to the virtual elimination of transfusion-related HIV transmission and dramatic reductions in perinatal transmission in many countries. Finally, the dramatic improvement in survival with ART has elevated the importance of early HIV detection and has fostered an emphasis on case finding, in addition to risk-reduction counseling.

In the United States, the Centers for Disease Control and Prevention (CDC) recommends that all patients aged 13–64 years seeking health care have routine HIV tests with opt-out consent. A variation of universal testing recommended by WHO, especially in developing countries, is provider-initiated testing and counseling (PITC). Although PITC implies pre-test counseling, it can be implemented with streamlined consent and it shifts the emphasis from a de facto requirement that patients recognize their risks and request HIV screening, to the provider to consider HIV testing in most or all patients. Widespread opt-out testing, similar to the CDC recommendations for the United States, has been promoted and apparently well accepted in Kenya and Uganda. A number of other innovative strategies to increase population-based HIV screening have been implemented in some sub-Saharan African countries, including services offered in the home or through mobile test facilities.

One of the most important developments in HIV prevention of the 2000s was documentation in three randomized controlled trials in Africa that circumcision of adult men reduces their risk of HIV by 50%. Social and infrastructural barriers exist to widespread implementation of male circumcision of young men or newborns, but substantial progress is being made in some countries. Increasing case detection and ART also have the potential to significantly reduce HIV transmission rates. Recent studies have also documented that pre-exposure prophylaxis (PrEP) with antiretroviral drugs administered either vaginally or orally can reduce HIV acquisition in women and MSM, respectively. Unfortunately, an effective vaccine against HIV has proved elusive, although promising research continues.

Complex bidirectional interactions exist between HIV and other STDs. These interactions contribute to susceptibility, transmission, and severity of both HIV and other STDs. Increased rates of GUD, particularly due to herpes, occur among individuals with HIV, apparently related in part to the degree of HIV-related immunologic impairment. Serologic evidence of syphilis has also been reported to be significantly more common among HIV-infected individuals in Africa, although this observation may reflect the behavioral determinants of both infections. Most important, there is a substantially elevated risk of HIV infection, typically by factors of 2-fold to 5-fold, in sexually active individuals with ulcerative or inflammatory STDs. These findings are supported by numerous studies suggesting that HIV shedding is increased in the presence of STDs, and that inflammatory cells recruited to urethritis, cervicitis, and GUD are especially susceptible to HIV if exposed.

Because of the high prevalence of genital herpes in all populations, particularly in geographic settings with high rates of HIV, infection with HSV-2 may account for up to half of all HIV infections (see Chap. 8). Successful treatment of HSV-2 infections, gonorrhea, and presumably other STDs reduces HIV shedding in genital secretions. Collectively, these observations suggested that treating STD-infected persons might help prevent HIV infection. Unfortunately, several controlled studies examining the effect of STD treatment failed to show reduced HIV transmission or incidence. It is important to note that most such studies were undertaken during mature HIV epidemics, in which sexual transmission may be relatively independent of STDs and high rates of partner change. At the individual level, successful treatment of STDs obviously is beneficial to the patient and his or her sex partners, and may help reduce HIV risk. And although antiherpetic therapy has failed to reduce HIV incidence in HSV-2-infected persons, it remains likely that successful primary prevention of HSV-2 infection and other inflammatory STDs would carry major benefits in HIV prevention. However, the quantitative contribution of STD control to HIV prevention at the population level remains to be defined.

Chlamydial Infection and Gonorrhea

According to WHO, an estimated 92 million new chlamydial infections and 62 million new cases of gonorrhea occur annually, making them the two most common bacterial STDs worldwide. Both pathogens are transmitted with relatively high efficiency, with 20 to 50% of unprotected vaginal sex exposures resulting in transmission if one partner is infected, complicating prevention and control. Except for urethral gonorrhea in men, most of these infections are subclinical, yet the morbidity they cause is substantial. Either infection commonly results in PID, whether overt or silent, with subsequent infertility, life-threatening ectopic pregnancy, and chronic pelvic pain. In pregnancy, either or both of these STDs can cause ophthalmia neonatorum (which in the case of gonorrhea can result in blindness), neonatal bronchitis and pneumonia, and postpartum endometritis (see Chaps. 3 and 4). In addition, both can cause acute epididymitis; chlamydial infection and perhaps gonorrhea can result in reactive arthritis; and gonorrhea can disseminate and lead to bacterial arthritis and, rarely, endocarditis or meningitis.

The global epidemiology of chlamydia and gonorrhea is notable for considerable variability in incidence over the past several decades. These trends have been influenced by improved diagnosis, increased screening, and improved clinical recognition, all of which can lead to elevated rates of reported infection that may belie actual declines. In principle, gonorrhea and chlamydial infections should be readily controllable, owing to availability of sensitive diagnostic tests and effective single-dose therapy. However, since the first use of sulfonamides and then penicillin for treatment of gonorrhea, control has been impaired by evolving antimicrobial resistance, now an especially difficult problem in resource-limited settings where antibiotic susceptibility monitoring is difficult and more effective treatment options may be unavailable. And while screening programs for the detection of asymptomatic chlamydia and gonorrhea are relatively widespread in some industrialized countries, few such programs exist in developing countries. Noninvasive screening strategies using NAATs on urine or self-collected vaginal swabs are potentially effective, but the required technical expertise and equipment render current NAATs impractical for widespread use in most developing countries. Development of rapid, inexpensive diagnostic tests for these infections may be especially important to facilitate improved prevention and control and may be more effective than syndromic management, as discussed above.

Syphilis

Syphilis has played an important role in human history and remains a highly morbid and frequent STD in many developing countries and in selected populations in industrialized ones (see Chap. 5). More than 12 million new cases of syphilis are estimated to occur annually, the large majority in southeast Asia and sub-Saharan Africa. In principle, syphilis is easily prevented and could readily be controlled with serological screening, single-dose penicillin therapy, and partner management. Indeed, in the mid- 1990s CDC declared an intention to eliminate syphilis from the United States, hoping to emulate the virtual elimination of the disease from China in the 1950s and 1960s. Unfortunately, syphilis has seen a remarkable resurgence in both countries, demonstrating the powerful influence of demography, behavior, and social dynamics in the face of effective biomedical interventions. Nevertheless, the incidence and prevalence of syphilis worldwide is now low in comparison with the mid-twentieth century, when penicillin was introduced. Prior to then, syphilis affected as much as 10% of the U.S. population and probably reached prevalence rates of 25% among some socioeconomically disadvantaged Americans. In addition, tertiary syphilis now is rare in industrialized countries and perhaps in many developing ones, probably due in part to frequent incidental treatment of undiagnosed infections when antibiotics are used for other indications.

More than most STDs, syphilis is heavily concentrated in population groups with especially large numbers of sex partners or anonymous partners, including commercial sex workers and some groups of MSM, particularly in industrialized countries. These high-risk populations have seen a remarkable resurgence of syphilis since in the mid-1990s in North America and western Europe. Poor access to health care, either overt or perceived, probably helped drive rising rates in Latinos in the southwestern United States during the late 2000s. Syphilis rates also increased in the late 2000s in heterosexual African Americans in several urban areas and the southeastern United States, at least in part because of some of the same social dynamics. Increasing rates of heterosexual transmission of syphilis have also led to widespread resurgence of the disease in China, where the disease apparently is concentrated in commercial sex workers, illicit drug users, and perhaps MSM. There are widespread impediments to control of syphilis in most or all developing countries, such as reliance on syndromic management of GUD, the absence of widespread screening, the need for injection penicillin therapy for reliable cure, and lack of resources to ensure treatment of sex partners. The seroprevalence of syphilis is as high as 10% in many areas of southern Africa, where the disease remains a major public health concern. The disease continues to carry strong stigma in most populations, sometimes rivaling that resulting from HIV/AIDS or tuberculosis.

The diagnosis of primary and sometimes secondary syphilis often rests on darkfield microcopy to detect *Treponema pallidum* in chancres and other lesions, but darkfield microscopy is technically demanding and is largely unavailable in both developing and industrialized countries. Therefore, serological testing is the mainstay of diagnosis and screening in all areas of the world (see Chap. 5). The recent development of *T. pallidum*-specific EIA and rapid point-of-care tests have revolutionized syphilis screening and diagnosis, in ways both good and bad. Case detection has been enhanced, especially in developing countries, but more positive results apparently are false or detect treated or inactive infection of little clinical or public health import. WHO syndromic management guidelines for GUD recommend treatment for presumed syphilis, as well as for chancroid, and the GUD algorithm is believed to have high sensitivity (70–100%) for the detection of primary syphilis and may have contributed to improved syphilis control in some settings. Nevertheless, improved diagnosis of syphilis is crucial for better control in both developing and developed countries. A sensitive NAAT has been developed but not marketed commercially; development of low-cost, low-technology tests for direct detection of *T. pallidum* is a high global health priority.

With tertiary syphilis now rare, congenital syphilis is generally regarded as the most serious manifestation of the disease and has a major impact on neonatal health worldwide, especially in developing countries. WHO estimates that 2 million pregnancies are affected by congenital syphilis each year, with a quarter of these pregnancies ending in miscarriage, stillbirth, or neonatal death. In addition to about 490,000 stillbirths and neonatal deaths annually, congenital syphilis is responsible for low birth weight or other serious disability in an additional 25% of affected infants. Despite widespread acceptance of guidelines that promote universal syphilis testing in pregnancy and treatment before delivery, adoption of these procedures has been suboptimal in many settings and seemingly ignored in some. Rapid diagnostic syphilis testing kits have been available for use in antenatal care settings in many developing countries since the late 2000s, and have resulted in an increase in the number of women tested and diagnosed with syphilis. Nevertheless, it is not clear that the proportion of infected women documented to actually receive effective treatment has significantly increased, especially where resource limitations have prevented use of appropriate drugs. For example, a survey of African countries where universal screening of pregnant women was adopted found that <40% of women attending antenatal care were screened and, if infected, received effective treatment. Improved prevention of congenital syphilis should be one of the world's top health priorities.

Herpes Simplex Virus Type 2 and Genital Human Papillomavirus Infections

Global interest and the focus of developing countries on HSV-2 and sexually transmitted human papillomavirus (HPV) infection has accelerated in recent years in response to increasing evidence of the important influence of the former on HIV transmission, and rising awareness of the burden of genital malignancies and improved opportunities for HPV prevention through immunization and improved screening. A study on behalf of WHO recently developed the first estimate of the global burden of HSV-2 infection. In 2003 the estimated prevalence was 536 million infected persons, about 8% of the world's population; the prevalence was about 20% in women aged 25–35 years. The annual incidence rate in the same year was estimated at 24 million persons. Regional variations are broad, with incidence estimates of 6 million new HSV-2 infections annually in sub-Saharan Africa, 5.3 million in eastern Asia, 1.1 million in North America, and 700,000 in western Europe. In addition to the impact of these epidemiologic trends on syndromic management of GUD, the special effect of HSV-2 on HIV transmission and the undoubtedly large (but unquantified) adverse effects on neonatal health make HSV-2 a major health burden in developing countries, and the prevalence undoubtedly continues to rise. Unfortunately, the challenges are great to prevention and control based on virologic and serologic testing. Incorporation of herpes treatment into GUD management may provide significant personal health benefit but is unlikely to have measurable population level impact on incidence or prevalence of genital HSV infections or their contribution to HIV transmission.

WHO estimates the global burden of cervical cancer at 510,000 new cases and 288,000 deaths annually, with >80% of cases occurring in developing countries. The estimated annual rate of about 40 cases of cervical cancer per 100,000 women is remarkably consistent in all countries in which economic and infrastructural barriers prevent routine screening with cervical cytology, and in industrialized countries in the era before cytology screening. In addition, the current rate of anal cancer caused by HPV in men who have sex with men is similar to that of cervical cancer in the absence of cytological screening. The etiologic role of specific HPV types has been reconfirmed multiple times in both developing and industrialized countries, and here too there is broad consistency, with 60–70% of cervical cancer and precancerous cervical disease attributed to HPV-16 or 18 in almost every country and population studied. The relative contributions of other HPV types to genital malignancies vary modestly, but the currently available bivalent and quadrivalent HPV vaccines have great potential for prevention in all countries, if cost and distribution impediments can be solved. The anticipated nonavalent vaccine, currently in clinical trials, probably will offer additional benefits in cancer prevention, covering up to 90% of cancer-causing HPV types in most countries. Increasing availability and declining costs of NAATs for high-risk HPV types, which can be performed on self-collected vaginal swabs, also will facilitate improved prevention in resource-limited countries. The burden of genital warts undoubtedly is also substantial in both developing and industrialized countries, but is appropriately a relatively low global health priority.

SUGGESTED READING

Aral SO, Holmes KK. The epidemiology of STIs and their social and behavioral determinants: industrialized and developing countries. Chapter 5 in KK Holmes, ed. *Sexually Transmitted Diseases*. 4th ed. New York, NY: McGraw-Hill; 2008:53-92. *A comprehensive summary of global STD trends.*

Dallabetta GA, et al. Prevention and control of STD and HIV infection in developing countries. Chapter 101 in KK Holmes, ed. *Sexually Transmitted Diseases*, 4th ed. New York, NY: McGraw-Hill, 2008:1957-76. *Summary of public health strategies to combat STDs in resource-limited settings.*

Lewis D. Modern management of genital ulcer disease—frappez fort et frappez vite [Editorial]. *Sex Transm Dis.* 2010;37(8):488-93. *A review and critique of current syndromic management guidelines for genital ulceration, with emphasis on the rising contribution of genital herpes.*

Looker KJ, et al. An estimate of the global prevalence and incidence of herpes simplex virus type 2 infection. *Bull World Health Organ.* 2008;86:805-12. *A comprehensive review of published data on HSV-2 seroprevalence and mathematical modeling to estimate worldwide and regional burden of HSV-2 infection.*

Wellings K, et al. Sexual behavior in context: a global perspective. *Lancet.* 2006;368:1706-28. *A review of sexual behavior patterns in 59 countries, with emphasis on demographic influences and implications for interventions to improve sexual health, including prevention of HIV and other STDs.*

World Health Organization. Guidelines for the management of sexually transmitted infections. Geneva, WHO, 2003. http://www.who.int/hiv/pub/sti/pub6/en/. Accessed August 1, 2010. *WHO's guidelines, including recommendations for syndromic diagnosis and management of STDs.*

World Health Organization. The global elimination of congenital syphilis: rationale and strategy for action. Geneva, WHO, 2007. http://www.who.int/reproductivehealth/publications/rtis/ 9789241595858/ en/index.html. Accessed August 1, 2010. A comprehensive review of the status of congenital syphilis globally and recommendations for prevention and control.

World Health Organization. Human papillomavirus infection and cervical cancer. Geneva, WHO, 2010. http://www.who.int/vaccine_research/diseases/hpv/en/. Accessed August 1, 2010. *Summary of global epidemiology of HPV and cervical cancer and prevention through immunization, with links to multiple WHO resources on related topics.*

• Section Two

Bacterial Sexually Transmitted Diseases

3

Chlamydial Infection

Chlamydia trachomatis is a small bacterium that invades eukaryotic cells and requires cell culture for isolation. Chlamydial infection is the most prevalent bacterial sexually transmitted disease (STD) in industrialized countries and perhaps worldwide; along with genital herpes and human papillomavirus (HPV) infection, it is one of the three most common STDs in the United States. Some serological variants (serovars) of *C. trachomatis* cause blinding trachoma, a continuing public health problem in some developing countries. Three serovars, designated L1, L2, and L3, cause lymphogranuloma venereum (LGV), one of the five classic venereal diseases (with gonorrhea, syphilis, chancroid, and granuloma inguinale). The LGV and trachoma serovars are uncommon in most populations in industrialized countries, but rectal infections with the L2 serovar have recently been resurgent among men who have sex with men (MSM). *Chlamydophila* (formerly *Chlamydia*) *pneumoniae* is a related respiratory pathogen that has been linked with coronary artery disease and atherosclerosis; it is not sexually transmitted.

In adults, the dominant manifestations of infection with the non–LGV serovars of *C. trachomatis* are nongonococcal urethritis, cervicitis, proctitis, and conjunctivitis, all of which commonly are mild and often asymptomatic. This clinical spectrum is similar to that of gonorrhea, but with less florid inflammatory symptoms and signs, a longer incubation period, and more frequent subclinical infection. Paradoxically, the outwardly mild nature of chlamydial infection may enhance the frequency of complications compared with gonorrhea, because treatment is often delayed and significant scarring (e.g., fallopian tube obstruction) can result from subclinical infection. The organism can be found in the upper genital tracts of most women with cervical infection, regardless of whether there are clinical manifestations of endometritis or salpingitis. Many women with tubal infertility or ectopic pregnancy following chlamydial infection have no past history of pelvic inflammatory disease (PID) or unexplained abdominal pain, indicating that subclinical salpingitis can result in tubal scarring. Repeat infection with *C. trachomatis* is associated with an elevated risk of complications, probably due to a vigorous anamnestic inflammatory response.

The development and widespread availability of nucleic acid amplification tests (NAATs) have markedly enhanced diagnosis. The prevalence of *C. trachomatis* in women declined modestly in several jurisdictions in the United States and western Europe following widespread introduction of systematic efforts to control chlamydial infections in the 1990s, based primarily on screening of sexually active women. However, most such geographic areas subsequently experienced substantial resurgences in prevalence in sexually active women, and probably in incidence, that could be attributed only in part to increased screening and use of improved diagnostic tests. It has been hypothesized that widespread screening and early treatment has had the paradoxical effect of enhancing the individual and perhaps population-level susceptibility to *C. trachomatis*, owing to reduced durable immunity that once resulted from more prolonged infections. The optimal approaches to preventing morbidity due to chlamydial infections, in particular the balance between further expansion of female screening, extending screening to sexually active men, and improved partner treatment, became the subject of debate in the late 2000s. Some experts have begun to question the utility of routine screening as a control strategy, but this stance is controversial, and the incidence of PID appears to be declining in the United States and the United Kingdom, plausibly the result of chlamydia prevention efforts based on screening. Routine screening of sexually active women and less extensive screening of males will continue in the foreseeable future.

EPIDEMIOLOGY

Incidence and Prevalence

- In the United States, 1.24 million cases reported in 2009; true estimated annual incidence 3–4 million
- Reported infections in the United States approximate 400 per 100,000 annually overall, 500–600 per 100,000 women, and 3,000 per 100,000 in females age 15–19 (equivalent to 3% of teen girls infected annually)
- True incidence rates are at least double these figures, due to underdiagnosis and underreporting
- Among women aged ≤25 years, prevalence averages ~5% in primary care practices and reproductive health clinics, 10–30% in STD clinics, and 5–10% in secondary school-based clinics, community centers, and social service sites
- Prevalence of urethral infection typically 5–10% in sexually active males aged 15–30 years; higher in MSM, including rectal infections
- LGV rare in the United States (reported cases <100/year in the 1990s) and western Europe; more common in some developing countries; recent increase in MSM

Transmission

- Exclusively by sexual contact or perinatally, except for transmission of trachoma serovars among children
- Pharyngeal infection and transmission by oral sex are rare, in contrast to gonorrhea
- LGV in MSM is transmitted by direct anal exposure, e.g., by hands or sex toys

Age

- Strong association with young age, probably due to both biological factors (e.g., physiologic cervical ectopy) and sexual behavior
- Peak incidence and prevalence age 15–19 years in females, 20–24 years in males

Sex

- More reported cases in women than men, because women are screened more frequently and many men are treated without diagnostic confirmation
- True M:F incidence ratio about 1:1

Sexual Orientation

- Common in MSM, but often undiagnosed due to high frequency of undetected rectal infection
- LGV occasionally causes severe proctitis in MSM
- Also common in some WSW without male partners, probably via shared vaginal secretions

Other Risk Factors

- In the United States, strong association with low socioeconomic and education levels and with African American or Hispanic race/ethnicity (as for most STDs)

HISTORY

Incubation Period

- Usually 1–3 weeks in those who develop symptoms; range 1 week to several months
- Many infections remain subclinical

Symptoms

- Males: Urethral discharge, often scant, and dysuria, usually mild, sometimes described as urethral itching or tingling
- Females: Vaginal discharge, dysuria, intermenstrual or postcoital vaginal bleeding, low abdominal pain; or other symptoms of urethritis, cervicitis, salpingitis, epididymitis, or conjunctivitis (see Chaps. 4, 15–20)

Epidemiologic and Exposure History

- Presence of STD risk factors and markers enhances risk, but infection is common in their absence
- Many infections persist for months and sometimes >1 year; recent sexual history often is a poor predictor of infection

PHYSICAL EXAMINATION

- Urethral, cervical, or anal discharge, usually mucoid or mucopurulent
- Edematous cervical ectopy in women
- Other signs of urethritis, cervicitis, salpingitis, proctitis, epididymitis, and other manifestations (see Chaps. 15–20)
- Examination is often normal

LABORATORY DIAGNOSIS

Identification of the Organism

- Test of choice is NAAT, including transcription-mediated amplification (TMA), e.g. Aptima, strand displacement assay (SDA), e.g. ProbeTec, or polymerase chain reaction (PCR), e.g. Amplicor
- NAAT sensitivity 90–95% for cervical, vaginal, or urethral swab, and urine specificity ≥99%, with rare false-positive results*
- TMA and SDA are reliable for rectal infection and recommended for testing MSM
- Some combination NAATs are designed to detect both *N. gonorrhoeae* and *C. trachomatis* in single specimens
- Culture detects 70–80% of cervical and urethral infections; substantial variability among laboratories
- Nonamplified DNA probe tests (e.g. Pace II) and assays to identify *C. trachomatis* antigens detect <80% of infections; approved only for urethral or cervical specimens; not recommended for routine use
- Currently available rapid (point of care) tests are insensitive and not recommended for routine use
- Pharyngeal infection is uncommon and no tests currently are approved or recommended for pharyngeal testing

Serology

- Microimmunofluorescence or complement fixation antibody tests useful in diagnosis of LGV (titer ≥1:128); sometimes used in evaluation of female infertility, but positive result does not necessarily indicate current infection
- Not recommended in other clinical settings

TREATMENT

Uncomplicated Infection

REGIMENS OF CHOICE

- Doxycycline 100 mg PO *bid* for 7 days
- Azithromycin 1.0 g PO, single dose

ALTERNATE REGIMENS

- Levofloxacin 500 mg PO once daily for 7 days
- Ofloxacin 300 mg PO *bid* for 7 days
- Erythromycin base 500 mg PO *qid* for 7 days (reduced efficacy)

---

* At the time of writing, PCR had lower specificity and caution is advised for use in low prevalence populations. However, manufacturers may modify currently available assays, with improved test performance.

Pregnant Women

- Azithromycin 1.0 g PO, single dose
- Amoxicillin 500 mg PO *qid* for 7–10 days

Lymphogranuloma Venereum

- Doxycycline 100 mg PO *bid* for 21 days
- Erythromycin base 500 mg PO *qid* for 21 days
- Azithromycin 1.0 g PO once weekly for 3 weeks (limited clinical experience)

Follow-up of Uncomplicated Infection

- Persistent or recurrent infection occurs within 3–6 months in 10–15% of treated patients
- Retest all patients 3–6 months after treatment (rescreening)
- Short-term test of cure (3–4 weeks):
  - When therapeutic compliance is uncertain
  - Pregnant women
  - Following erythromycin or other nonstandard treatment
  - Do not retest with NAAT <3 weeks after treatment, due to possible persistence of chlamydial DNA despite successful eradication

MANAGEMENT OF SEX PARTNERS

- All sex partners in preceding month, as well as all likely source partners, should be tested for *C. trachomatis* and treated (without awaiting test results)
- Expedited partner treatment (EPT) (e.g., patient-delivered partner treatment) is indicated when partner compliance with direct health care is uncertain
  - EPT is recommended by some experts as management of choice for all partners
  - When practical, partners managed with EPT still should be examined, tested, and counseled

PREVENTION

Counseling

- Emphasize importance of preventing future infections, due to enhanced risk of complications, especially in women
- Encourage monogamy, condoms, selection of sex partners at low risk, and avoidance of concurrency (overlapping partnerships)
- Describe higher risk of HIV infection in persons with bacterial STD

Screening

- Screening sexually active young women is central to prevention
- Routinely test all sexually active women ≤20 years old

- Routinely test women 21–30 years old if ≥1 sex partner, new partner, or partner with symptoms of urethritis
- Sexually active teen boys and young men (≤30 years old) should be routinely screened when practical
- Urine or self-collected swab testing by NAAT permits screening when genital examination impractical
- Routine rectal screening of MSM who participate in receptive anal intercourse
- Screen all pregnant women

Rescreening

- Routinely retest all patients 3–6 months after treatment, and/or whenever the patient returns for routine health care
- 10–20% of infected persons have recurrent or persistent infection at 3–6 months due to reinfection, delayed treatment failure, or poor therapeutic compliance

Reporting

- Report cases as required by local regulations

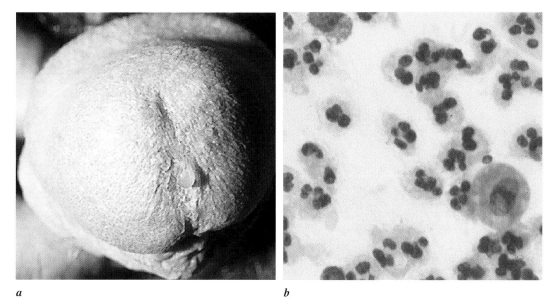

a   *b*

3–1. Nongonococcal urethritis due to *Chlamydia trachomatis*. *a*. Mucopurulent urethral discharge. Gram-stained urethral smear showing PMNs without ICGND. Compare with Figs. 4–1, 4–3*b*, 4–6, 4–8, and 18–3*b*.

CASE

Patient Profile Age 19, single heterosexual college sophomore

History Began new sexual relationship 6 weeks earlier; prior partnership ended 2 months ago; 3 weeks' intermittent urethral discharge without dysuria; referred by his new partner after she had positive screening test for *C. trachomatis*

Examination Mucopurulent discharge expressed by urethral compression

Differential Diagnosis Nongonococcal urethritis (NGU); probably chlamydial based on exposure history; gonococcal, trichomonal, and herpetic urethritis possible but unlikely

Laboratory Urethral Gram stain showed 10–15 polymorphonuclear neutrophils (PMNs) per 1000 × field, without ICGND; NAATs for *C. trachomatis* (positive) and *N. gonorrhoeae* (negative); VDRL and HIV antibody test (both negative)

Diagnosis Chlamydial NGU

Treatment Azithromycin 1.0 g PO, single dose, directly observed

Sex Partner Management Offered expedited partner treatment (EPT) with azithromycin and cefixime for former girlfriend, but patient declined ("I don't see her anymore"); advised to abstain from sex with current partner until 1 week and symptoms resolved

Follow-up Advised to return in 3 months for rescreening by urine NAAT, and counseled to convey same advice to partner

Comment Mild symptoms resulted in delayed care (3 weeks) until partner's chlamydial infection was diagnosed

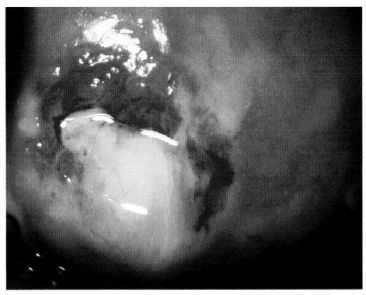

3–2. Mucopurulent cervicitis due to *Chlamydia trachomatis*. (*Courtesy of Claire E. Stevens.*)

CASE

Patient Profile Age 17, high school junior

History Asymptomatic; presented to a public reproductive health clinic for refill of her oral contraceptive prescription; sexually active for 6 weeks with a single male partner, a local college student; a prior relationship, with a high school classmate, ended 2 months earlier

Examination Mucopurulent exudate emanating from cervical os; small area of edematous cervical ectopy; swab-induced endocervical bleeding

Differential Diagnosis Mucopurulent cervicitis; consider *C. trachomatis*, *N. gonorrhoeae*, *Mycoplasma genitalium*

Laboratory Cervical Gram-stained smear showed many PMNs, without ICGND; vaginal fluid pH 4.0 with negative KOH amine odor test; no yeast, clue cells, or trichomonads seen on KOH and saline wet mounts; cervical NAATs for *C. trachomatis* (positive) and *N. gonorrhoeae* (negative); serologic tests for syphilis and HIV (negative)

Diagnosis Mucopurulent cervicitis due to *C. trachomatis*

Treatment Azithromycin 1.0 g PO, single dose, directly observed

Follow-up Advised to return 3 months for rescreening by NAAT on self-collected vaginal swab

Sex Partner Management Offered and accepted EPT with azithromycin for current partner, who was away at university; referred former partner to clinic, tested positive for *C. trachomatis* and treated

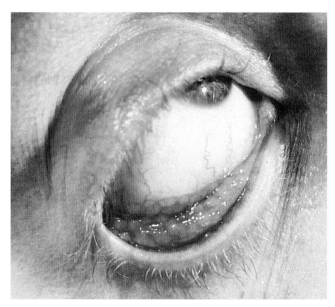

3–3. Chlamydial conjunctivitis (compare with gonococcal conjunctivitis, Fig. 4–3*a*).

CASE

Patient Profile Age 22, female flight attendant

History Mild itching of eyes for 2–3 weeks; boyfriend was treated a month earlier for "urinary tract infection"; they continued unprotected vaginal and oral sex following his treatment; no other sex partners in the past year

Examination Conjunctiva showed hypertrophied, "cobblestone" appearance, slight erythema; genital examination normal, including cervix

Differential Diagnosis Conjunctivitis due to *C. trachomatis, N. gonorrhoeae, Haemophilus influenzae*, other pyogenic bacteria, viruses, or allergy; rule out cervical *C. trachomatis* infection

Laboratory Gram-stained conjunctival smear showed few mononuclear cells, rare PMNs, and no bacteria; *C. trachomatis* indentified by NAAT from conjunctival and cervical swabs; bacterial culture of conjunctiva negative for pathogens

Diagnosis Chlamydial conjunctivitis and asymptomatic cervical chlamydial infection

Treatment Doxycycline 100 mg PO *bid* for 7 days

Follow-up Advised to return after 3 months for rescreening with NAAT

Sex Partner Management Advised to refer her partner for reevaluation of probable NGU, suspected to have been misdiagnosed as urinary tract infection (UTI); patient was skeptical partner would attend and was provided EPT with azithromycin 1.0 g

Comment Compare with gonococcal conjunctivitis, Fig. 4–3; probably acquired either through autoinoculation from genital infection or by orogenital exposure; normal cervix and absence of genital symptoms are typical of chlamydial infection

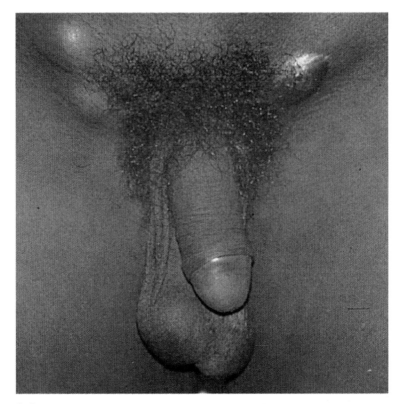

3–4. Lymphogranuloma venereum. Note separation of right lymph nodes by the inguinal ligament ("groove sign"). The left inguinal node had ruptured spontaneously. (*Courtesy of Professor Olu Osoba.*)

CASE

Patient Profile Age 27, unmarried man who immigrated from Ethiopia 3 weeks earlier; multiple female commercial sex partners

History Painful swellings in groin for 3 weeks; draining pus from left side for 1 week

Examination Inguinal lymphadenopathy bilaterally, with firm, moderately tender nodes, 1.5–3 cm in diameter; left inguinal node had central softening and an overlying eschar; right nodes were divided by the inguinal ligament ("groove sign"); no urethral discharge, genital lesions, or skin rash

Differential Diagnosis LGV, pyogenic infection, cat-scratch disease; liquefaction and drainage make syphilis and herpes unlikely; rule out tuberculous lymphadenitis, lymphoma, and HIV-related opportunistic diseases

Laboratory Urethral NAATs for *N. gonorrhoeae* and *C. trachomatis* (both negative); syphilis and HIV serology (both negative); aspirate of left inguinal node yielded scant pus, without organisms on Gram stain; few *Staphylococcus epidermidis* isolated, negative NAAT for *C. trachomatis;* chlamydia/LGV complement fixation test titer 1:1,024

Diagnosis Lymphogranuloma venereum

Treatment Doxycycline 100 mg orally *bid* for 3 weeks

Follow-up Repeated needle aspiration of left inguinal node (3 times over 8 days); repeat syphilis and HIV serology after 3 months (negative)

Sex Partner Management Patient denied identifiable sex partners

Comment Absence of detectable cutaneous primary lesion or urethritis is typical of LGV; division of involved lymph nodes by the inguinal ligament ("groove sign") is classic but seen in a minority of cases; repeated needle aspiration of fluctuant nodes may help prevent spontaneous rupture and secondary infection; currently the most common clinical presentation of LGV in industrialized countries is proctitis in MSM

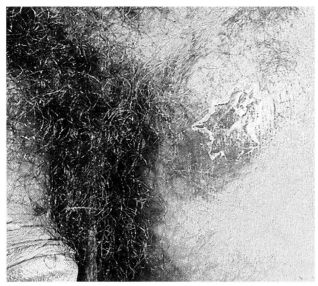

a

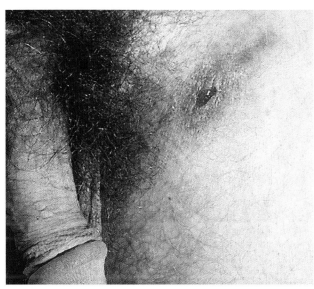

b

3–5. Probable lymphogranuloma venereum. *a.* Fluctuant femoral lymphadenopathy with intense overlying cutaneous erythema and nonspecific exfoliation at presentation. *b.* Improvement after 10 days treatment with doxycycline 100 mg orally *bid.* Femoral involvement is atypical in LGV and *C. trachomatis* was not isolated by culture from lymph node aspirate or urethra; NAAT was not available. However, the LGV complement fixation titer was reactive at a titer of 1:512. Papular genital warts also are present on penile shaft.

SUGGESTED READING

Gaydos C, et al. Laboratory aspects of screening men for *Chlamydia trachomatis* in the new millennium. *Sex Transm Dis.* 2008;35(Suppl):S40-4. *In addition to screening men, this review is a good introduction to available NAATs for chlamydial infection.*

Gottlieb SL, et al, eds. Introduction: natural history and immunobiology of *Chlamydia trachomatis* genital infection and implications for chlamydia control. *J Infect Dis.* 2010;201(Suppl 2):S85-7. *The introductory article to 11 reviews of the biology, clinical manifestations, prevention and control of sexually transmitted chlamydial infections.*

McLean CA, et al. Treatment of lymphogranuloma venereum. *Clin Infect Dis.* 2007;44(Suppl 3):S147-52. *Review of the data in support of CDC's 2006 STD treatment guidelines.*

Oakeshott P, et al. Randomised controlled trial of screening for *Chlamydia trachomatis* to prevent pelvic inflammatory disease: the POPI (prevention of pelvic infection) trial. *BMJ.* 2010;340:c1642. *A study showing modest benefit of chlamydia screening in PID prevention and a useful introduction to public health chlamydia prevention strategies.*

Scholes D, et al. Prevention of pelvic inflammatory disease by screening for cervical chlamydial infection. *N Engl J Med.* 1996;334:1362-6. *A prospective study documenting reduced incidence of symptomatic PID in women screened for chlamydial infection; a central underpinning of chlamydia prevention strategies.*

Schwebke JR, et al. Re-evaluating the treatment of nongonococcal urethritis: emphasizing emerging pathogens—a randomized clinical trial. *Clin Infect Dis.* 2011;52:163-70. *This multicenter trial raised questions about the efficacy of azithromycin for chlamydial NGU, with a 77% cure rate, compared with 95% for doxycycline.*

Stamm WE. *Chlamydia trachomatis* infections. Chapter 29 in KK Holmes, et al., eds. *Sexually Transmitted Diseases.* 4th ed. New York, NY: McGraw-Hill, 2008:775-93. *A comprehensive, extensively referenced state-of-the-art review.*

White JA. Manifestations and management of lymphogranuloma venereum. *Curr Opin Infect Dis.* 2009;22:57-66. *A succinct review of recently emergent LGV in men who have sex with men.*

4

Gonorrhea

Gonorrhea is among the most common and most widely recognized sexually transmitted diseases (STDs) throughout the world. It is one of the five classical venereal diseases, with syphilis, chancroid, lymphogranuloma venereum, and donovanosis (granuloma inguinale). *Neisseria gonorrhoeae*, a Gram-negative diplococcus that in clinical material typically appears within polymorphonuclear leukocytes (PMNs), primarily infects the mucosal surfaces of the urethra or endocervix and secondarily those of the rectum and pharynx. Conjunctivitis can occur by exposure to infected secretions, including auto-inoculation in patients with genital infection. Ascending infection in women results in gonococcal pelvic inflammatory disease (PID), the most common complication and an important cause of female infertility. Bacteremic dissemination causes a characteristic arthritis–dermatitis syndrome or septic arthritis, and rarely bacterial endocarditis or meningitis. Other complications are acute epididymitis and, in infants born to infected mothers, conjunctivitis (gonococcal ophthalmia neonatorum) that can result in corneal scarring and consequent blindness. Transmission occurs almost exclusively through sexual or perinatal exposure.

Evolution of antibiotic-resistant *N. gonorrhoeae* worldwide has rendered ineffective formerly recommended regimens of the sulfonamides, penicillins, tetracyclines, and fluoroquinolones. Ceftriaxone remains active, but relative resistance to cefixime and other oral cephalosporins has evolved in parts of Asia and likely will spread and rare ceftriaxone-resistant strains have been isolated in east Asia. Eventual dissemination of ceftriaxone resistant gonococci remains a distinct possibility, and the recommended dose of ceftriaxone has been raised from 125 to 250 mg. It has long been recommended that single-dose treatment with a cephalosporin or other recommended antibiotic be followed by azithromycin or doxycycline to treat simultaneous chlamydial infection, present in 15–30% of persons with gonorrhea. In order to help retard evolution of antibiotic resistance in *N. gonorrhoeae*, such dual therapy is now recommended by the Centers for Disease Control and Prevention (CDC) and other experts even if simultaneous chlamydial infection has been excluded. Clinicians should remain alert to possible frequent modifications in recommended treatments. As for chlamydial infection, 10–20% of patients with gonorrhea have persistent or recurrent infection when retested 3–6 months after treatment, and all patients with gonorrhea should be routinely rescreened for both *N. gonorrhoeae* and *C. trachomatis*.

EPIDEMIOLOGY

Incidence and Prevalence

- In the United States, reported cases fell 78% from peak 1,013,436 (454 per 100,000 population) in 1978 to 301,174 cases (99 per 100,000) in 2009; true total probably is double the reported cases, i.e. ~600,000 infections annually

- Global incidence highly variable; generally low in industrialized countries, but widely underreported

- European Union had total 29,000 reported cases in 2007; <15 per 100,000 in all western European countries

- WHO estimates 170 million cases per year worldwide

- Strong associations in all societies with low socioeconomic status, population migration, societal disruption, armed conflict, commercial sex, and reduced access to health care

- Prevalence varies widely:
  - Typically 5–20% of patients in many urban STD clinics and some corrections facilities
  - Generally <1% of sexually active women in private physicians' offices and most reproductive health clinics
  - Usually 5–10% of men who have sex with men (MSM) seeking care for STD

Transmission

- Most cases are acquired by vaginal or anal intercourse; estimated transmission risk per unprotected exposure 20–50%

- Less efficient transmission by fellatio, especially from pharynx to genitals, but explains most pharyngeal infections in women and MSM and up to 40% of urethral gonorrhea in MSM

- Least efficient by cunnilingus, accounting for rare pharyngeal infection

Age

- All ages susceptible

- In the United States, ~80% of cases occur in females aged 15–29 years and males aged 15–34 years

Sex

- In the United States, reported cases in females slightly outnumber those in men (ratio 1.2 to 1 in 2009), owing to more frequent screening of women; actual case rates are probably similar in heterosexual men and women, elevated in MSM

- Distribution by sex varies with success of case-finding in asymptomatic women, frequency of commercial sex, and local rates in MSM

Sexual Orientation

- Rising rates in cases of MSM in industrialized countries during 1998–2009

- Annual rate in MSM is several times higher than in heterosexuals
  - In King County, Washington, estimated 2009 annual rate per 100,000 was 28 times higher in MSM (1,105 per 100,000) than heterosexual men (40 per 100,000)

- ○ Similar differentials probably are the norm, but not systematically analyzed in most geographic areas
- Exchange of vaginal secretions can transmit gonorrhea in WSW

Race/Ethnicity

- In the United States, compared with whites, reported rates in 2009 were 20 times higher in African Americans (27 vs. 556 per 100,000), twice as high in persons of Hispanic ethnicity, 4 times higher in native Americans, and one-third lower in persons of Asian or Pacific Island ancestry
- Race and ethnicity are indirect markers of socioeconomic status, access to health care, education, and sexual network patterns (see Chap. 1)

Other Risk Markers

- Unmarried
- Lower educational and socioeconomic status
- Illicit drug use
- Commercial sex
- Previous gonorrhea

HISTORY

Incubation Period

- Typically 2 to 5 days for urethritis in men
- 5–10 days in women with anogenital gonorrhea
- 1–5% of urethral infections in men and 20–40% of cervical infections remain subclinical for prolonged periods
- Most rectal and pharyngeal infections are asymptomatic

Symptoms

- Urethritis in males: urethral discharge, often copious; dysuria, sometimes severe
- Uncomplicated genital infection in females: any combination of increased vaginal discharge, dysuria, intermenstrual bleeding (sometimes postcoital), low abdominal pain, or other symptoms of urethritis, cervicitis, salpingitis, epididymitis, or conjunctivitis (see Chaps. 3, 15, 16, 18–20)
- Rectal infection (proctitis): usually asymptomatic; symptomatic cases usually present with any combination of anal discharge (often described as exudate on feces), anal pruritus, occasionally tenesmus, rectal bleeding (see Chap. 21)
- Pharyngeal infection: usually asymptomatic; occasionally mild sore throat; rare exudative pharyngitis
- Complicated infections: main symptoms are low abdominal pain (in women), testicular pain and swelling, polyarthralgia, joint swelling, skin lesions, conjunctival pain and discharge, constitutional symptoms

Epidemiologic and Exposure History

- Uncommon in absence of behavioral risk factors and demographic markers (unlike chlamydial infection)
- Most patients acknowledge new sex partner or partner known to have other partners in preceding 1–2 months

PHYSICAL EXAMINATION

Urethritis in Males

- Urethral discharge, usually overt; sometimes demonstrable only by "milking" urethra
- Discharge usually is frankly purulent, i.e. opaque, white or yellow in color; sometimes mucoid or mucopurulent
- Occasional meatal erythema
- Rarely penile edema or lymphangitis
- May be normal in men with subclinical infection

Urogenital Infection in Women

- Purulent or mucopurulent endocervical exudate; other signs of mucopurulent cervicitis (see Chap. 18)
- Sometimes purulent exudate expressible from the urethra, periurethral (Skene's) glands, or Bartholin gland duct
- Uterine, adnexal, or abdominal tenderness or mass, suggesting PID (see Chap. 20)
- Often entirely normal

Rectal Infection

- External examination usually normal
- Anoscopy may show mucosal erythema, punctate bleeding, purulent exudate (see Chap. 21)

Pharyngeal Infection

- Usually normal
- Rarely erythema, purulent exudate, cervical lymphadenopathy

Localized and Systemic Complications

- Abdominal tenderness, pelvic adnexal tenderness, pelvic mass (see Chap. 20)
- Testicular tenderness, enlargement (usually unilateral) (see Chap. 16)
- Tenosynovitis, joint tenderness, and erythema
- Skin lesions: petechiae, papules, pustules (sometimes hemorrhagic)
- Conjunctival erythema, purulent exudate

LABORATORY DIAGNOSIS

Gram-Stained Smear*

- PMNs with intracellular gram-negative diplococci (ICGND); test performance depends substantially on skills and experience of examiner

---

*Methylene blue and other monochromatic stains are frequently used in some settings and have performance characteristics similar to Gram stain.

- Highly accurate in symptomatic male urethritis: ≥90% sensitive, ≥95% specific (i.e., false-negative and false-positive results are rare)
- Insensitive for cervical, rectal, or asymptomatic urethral infection, detecting <50% of cases; but highly specific with experienced observer
- Not useful for pharyngeal infection

Nucleic Acid Amplification Tests

- NAAT is usual test of choice, including transcription-mediated amplification (TMA), e.g. Aptima, strand displacement assay (SDA), e.g. ProbeTec, or polymerase chain reaction (PCR), e.g. Amplicor[†]
- Combination NAATs detect both *N. gonorrhoeae* and *C. trachomatis* in single specimens
- NAAT detects 90–95% of infections in genital secretions (cervical, vaginal, or urethral swab, or urine) and rarely are false-positive
- Rectal and pharyngeal infection: TMA appears reliable

Culture

- Isolation on selective growth medium; preserves isolate for antimicrobial susceptibility testing or for confirmation for medicolegal purposes, when needed
- Sensitivity: urethra ≥95%; cervix 80–90%; rectum 70–80%; pharynx 60–70%

Other Tests

- Nonamplified DNA probe tests (e.g., Pace II) and antigen detection assays are less sensitive than NAAT; false-positive results may be common in low-prevalence settings
- Only culture and NAAT are recommended to detect rectal or pharyngeal gonorrhea

TREATMENT

Principles

- Penicillin resistance: Resistant *N. gonorrhoeae* is prevalent worldwide, both plasmid-mediated β-lactamase production and chromosomal
- Fluoroquinolones: Resistance is now prevalent worldwide
- Cephalosporins: Clinically significant resistance to oral cephalosporins has appeared in parts of Asia; to date uncommon elsewhere but increasing spread is anticipated; ceftriaxone resistance may be increasing but currently rare
- Recommended single-dose regimens are ≥95% effective for urethral, cervical, and rectal infections
- Recommended regimens have variable and generally lower efficacy for pharyngeal infection

---

[†]At the time of writing, PCR and SDA had lower specificity than TMA; caution is advised for use in low-prevalence populations. However, manufacturers may modify available assays, with improved test performance.

- Treat all gonorrhea patients with azithromycin or doxycycline as recommended for *C. trachomatis* infection
- Dual therapy also may help retard selection of antibiotic-resistant *N. gonorrhoeae* and should be employed even when chlamydial infection has been excluded

Uncomplicated Genital or Rectal Gonorrhea in Adults

Regimen of Choice

- Ceftriaxone 250 mg IM (single dose) and *either* azithromycin 1.0 g PO (single dose) *or* doxycycline 100 mg PO *bid* for 7 days

Primary Alternative if Ceftriaxone Cannot Be Given

- Cefixime 400 mg PO (single dose) *and* azithromycin or doxycycline, as above

Other Alternative Regimens

- Cefpodoxime 400 mg PO (single dose) *and* azithromycin or doxycycline, as above; *or*
- Cefuroxime 1.0 g PO (single dose) *and* azithromycin or doxycycline, as above; *or*
- Azithromycin 2.0 g PO (single dose)

Pharyngeal Gonorrhea

- Ceftriaxone *and* azithromycin or doxycycline, as above
- Other single-dose regimens have reduced efficacy when given alone, but probably are reliable in combination with azithromycin or doxycycline

Pregnant Women

- Ceftriaxone or cefixime as above, *and* azithromycin 1.0 g PO
- Azitrhomycin 2.0 g PO (single dose) if cephalosporins contraindicated
- If azithromycin not available, use ceftriaxone or cefixime, *and* either amoxicillin or erythromycin as recommended for *C. trachomatis* during pregnancy (see Chap. 3)

Disseminated Gonococcal Infection

- Ceftriaxone 1.0 g IM or IV every 24 hours until improved, then cefixime 400 mg PO *bid* to complete 7 days total therapy
- A fluoroquinolone (e.g., ciprofloxacin) may given initially or to complete 7 days therapy, if susceptibility testing demonstrates sensitivity
- For endocarditis, give parenteral cephalosporin therapy for 4 to 6 weeks

Gonococcal Conjunctivitis in Adults

- Ceftriaxone 1.0 g IM, single dose

Follow-up

- Retest all patients 3–6 months after treatment (rescreening); 10–20% of patients have either reinfection or delayed treatment failure

- Test of cure at 3–4 weeks:
  - If therapeutic compliance is uncertain
  - Pregnant women
  - Following nonstandard treatment
  - Do not retest with NAAT sooner than 3 weeks after treatment, due to possible persistence of gonococcal DNA despite successful eradication

MANAGEMENT OF SEX PARTNERS

- All sex partners in preceding month, as well as all likely source partners, should be tested for *N. gonorrhoeae* and treated (without awaiting test results)
- Expedited partner treatment (EPT) (e.g., patient-delivered partner treatment) is indicated whenever partner compliance with direct health care is uncertain
  - EPT is recommended by some experts as management of choice for all partners
  - When practical, partners managed with EPT also should be examined, tested, and counseled

PREVENTION

Counseling

- Emphasize importance of preventing future infections and ensuring treatment of partners
- Encourage monogamy, condoms, selection of sex partners at low risk, and avoidance of concurrency (overlapping partnerships)
- Emphasize the substantially elevated risk of HIV infection in persons with gonorrhea
- Address lifestyle issues that are common risk markers for gonorrhea, including commercial sex, substance abuse, concurrency, abusive relationships, sexual coercion

Screening

- Formal recommendations for gonorrhea screening are lacking in the United States, but testing for *N. gonorrhoeae* is the norm when screening for chlamydia
- Routinely test women in population groups and settings with high rates of gonorrhea whenever they seek health care
- Screening men for urethral gonorrhea is of uncertain value, because asymptomatic urethral infection is rare
- Test MSM for rectal and pharyngeal infection, depending on sites exposed

Reporting

- Report cases to health authorities according to local regulations

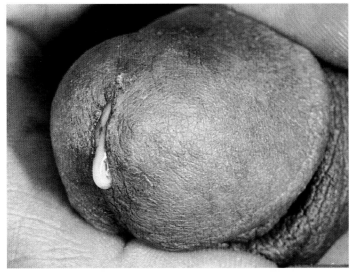
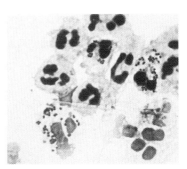

a   *b*

4–1. Gonococcal urethritis. *a.* Purulent urethral discharge. *b.* Gram-stained smear showing intracellular gram-negative diplococci.

CASE

Patient Profile Age 22, carwash attendant

History Urethral discharge for 1 day, mild dysuria; vaginal intercourse with a new female partner 4 days earlier and with regular girlfriend 2 days ago

Examination Copious purulent urethral discharge

Differential Diagnosis Gonorrhea, nongonococcal urethritis

Laboratory PMNs with ICGND on urethral smear; urethral NAATs for *N. gonorrhoeae* and *C. trachomatis* (both positive); VDRL and HIV serology (both negative)

Diagnosis Gonococcal urethritis (with chlamydial infection)

Treatment Cefixime 400 mg PO plus azithromycin 1.0 g PO (both single dose, directly observed)

Follow-up Advised to return in 3 months for rescreening with urine NAAT for *N. gonorrhoeae* and *C. trachomatis*

Sex Partner Management Advised to refer partners; patient agreed to refer his new partner and opted for EPT for his regular partner, with cefixime and azithromycin

Comment Up to 25% of heterosexual men with gonorrhea also have urethral *C. trachomatis* infection

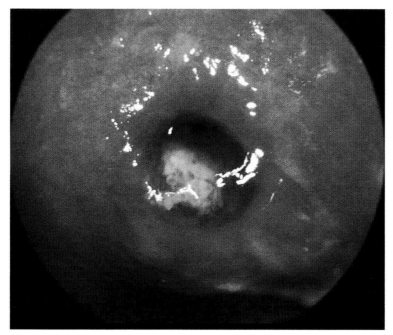

4–2. Gonococcal cervicitis, with scant purulent exudate in os. (*Courtesy of King K. Holmes, M.D., Ph.D.*)

CASE

Patient Profile Age 18, new partner of preceding patient

History Asymptomatic; no other partners in past 4 months; skin rash after receiving penicillin during childhood

Examination Mucopurulent cervical exudate; otherwise normal

Differential Diagnosis Mucopurulent cervicitis; contact and referral history suggests gonorrhea; 20–30% probability of concomitant chlamydial infection

Laboratory Gram stain of cervical exudate showed PMNs without ICGND; cervical NAATs for *N. gonorrhoeae* and *C. trachomatis* (both positive); VDRL and HIV serology negative

Diagnosis Gonococcal cervicitis (with chlamydial infection)

Treatment Cefixime 400 mg PO, single dose, directly observed; plus azithromycin 1.0 g PO, single dose

Follow-up Advised to return in 3 months for rescreening with urine NAAT for *N. gonorrhoeae* and *C. trachomatis*

Sex Partner Management The only partner at risk had been treated

Comment Although allergic cross reactivity can occur between penicillin and cephalosporins, it is uncommon and oral cefixime (or IM ceftriaxone) is considered safe by most experts

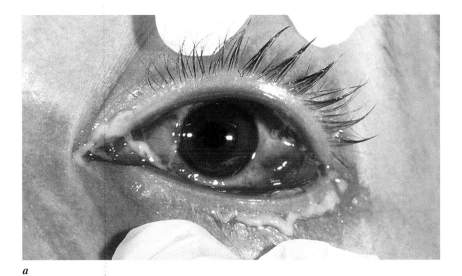

a

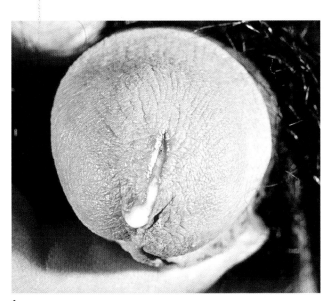

b

4–3. *a.* Gonococcal conjunctivitis; compare with chlamydial conjunctivitis (see Fig. 3–3). *b.* Purulent discharge in gonococcal urethritis.

CASE

Patient Profile Age 33, male, computer programmer, MSM, HIV positive, on antiretroviral therapy

History Urethral discharge for 3 days; increasingly severe left eye pain and photophobia for 2 days; visited an urgent care clinic 1 day earlier for eye pain, treated with eye drops; one regular sex partner who also has HIV; patient suspects partner has other partners

Examination Marked conjunctival erythema, copious purulent exudate, subconjunctival hemorrhage; purulent urethral discharge

Differential Diagnosis Urethritis, probably gonorrhea; rule out chlamydial infection and NGU; purulent conjunctivitis, rule out gonorrhea, other pyogenic infections, herpes, *C. trachomatis*

Laboratory PMNs with ICGND in both conjunctival and urethral exudate; both culture and NAAT from both sites positive for *N. gonorrhoeae*; urethral and conjunctival NAAT negative for *C. trachomatis* and negative by culture for herpes simplex virus (HSV); rectal NAAT and pharyngeal culture negative for *N. gonorrhoeae*; rectal NAAT negative for *C. trachomatis*; VDRL negative

Diagnosis Gonococcal urethritis and conjunctivitis

Treatment Ceftriaxone 250 mg IM, single dose, followed by doxycycline 100 mg PO *bid* for 7 days

Follow-up Scheduled to return after 2 days to assess conjunctivitis, which had markedly improved

Sex Partner Management Patient notified his partner, who was treated by his private physician

Comment Compare with chlamydial conjunctivitis (see Fig. 3–3); conjunctivitis may have resulted from autoinoculation from patient's urethral infection, or from direct oropharyngeal exposure; some HIV-infected MSM continue high-risk sex or have partners who do so

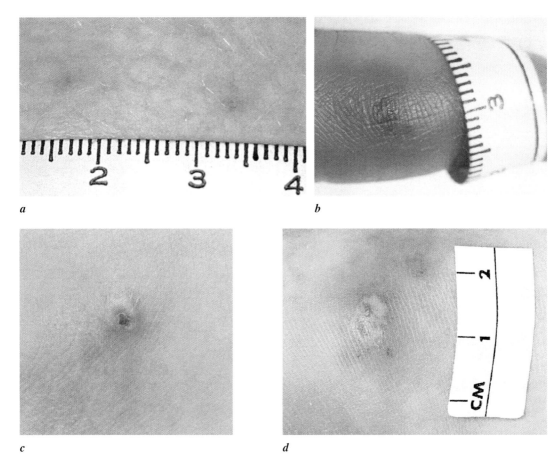

a

b

c

d

4–4. Skin lesions in gonococcal arthritis–dermatitis syndrome. a. Early papular lesions of forearm. b. Hemorrhagic lesion of finger. c. Pustule with central eschar. d. Large hemorrhagic pustule of foot. (Parts a and b are from the case described below. Parts c and d are from two other patients.) Lesions typically begin as nonspecific papules or petechiae, and then progress to pustules, often with a hemorrhagic component. The rulers in parts a, b, and d are metric.

CASE

Patient Profile Age 22, female, exotic dancer in a strip club

History Generalized aching of arms and legs and "red bumps" on all four extremities for 2 days; overt pain of several joints for 1 day; intermittent vaginal discharge for several months without recent change; currently menstruating; refused to give information about sex partners or sexual practices in connection with her work

Examination Afebrile; 15–20 papular, pustular, and hemorrhagic skin lesions on extremities; slight erythema and edema over left wrist, extending to dorsum of hand; pain on range of motion of left ankle, without visible abnormality; moderate effusion of right knee, with 20 mL slightly cloudy, straw-colored fluid withdrawn by needle aspiration; menstrual blood in vaginal vault, genital examination otherwise normal; normal cardiac examination

Differential Diagnosis Disseminated gonococcal infection (arthritis–dermatitis syndrome); also consider reactive arthritis, hepatitis B prodrome, other immune-complex syndromes, meningococcemia, bacterial endocarditis, acute rheumatic fever, systemic lupus erythematosus, and other etiologies of acute arthritis

Laboratory Synovial fluid contained 8,500 leukocytes per mm^3, 80% PMNs, no crystals, no bacteria observed by Gram stain; in pre-NAAT era, cultures for *N. gonorrhoeae* from cervix, anal canal, pharynx, synovial fluid, and blood (×3); cervical culture for *C. trachomatis* (negative); CBC showed 12,400 leukocytes, 80% PMNs, otherwise normal; chemistry panel normal, including liver function tests; VDRL, HIV, and hepatitis B serologies negative; *N. gonorrhoeae* isolated from cervix and pharynx; other cultures negative

Diagnosis Disseminated gonococcal infection with arthritis–dermatitis syndrome

Treatment Ceftriaxone 1.0 g IM, repeated 1 day later; then ofloxacin 300 mg PO *bid* for 8 days (10 days total therapy)

Follow-up Followed daily for 3 days till completion of therapy; arthritis improved within 1 day and resolved by day 5; skin lesions were healed at 10 days

Sex Partner Management At first follow-up visit, health department counselor reinterviewed patient, without success in identifying partners

Comment Onset of DGI (disseminated gonococcal infection) during or near menses is typical. Many patients, like this one, are afebrile; high fever may be an indication for IV therapy and usually hospitalization. Synovial fluid cultures usually are negative in arthritis–dermatitis stage, but often positive if overt septic arthritis supervenes. Blood cultures may be positive or negative. Careful cardiac examination and close follow-up are indicated for first 2–3 days to evaluate for gonococcal endocarditis. This patient presented before fluoroquinolone-resistant *N. gonorrhoeae* was prevalent, and ofloxacin was selected for completion of therapy because of efficacy against both *N. gonorrhoeae* and *C. trachomatis*. DGI is associated with particular gonococcal strains that are currently uncommon in most geographic areas.

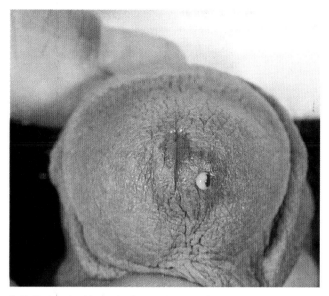

4–5. Periurethral furuncle due to *N. gonorrhoeae*. Patient presented with history of "pimple" at tip of penis, draining intermittently for 6 weeks, without urethral discharge or dysuria. Pathogenesis may have been infection of a sebaceous gland or other preexisting skin lesion. Gram stain of exudate showed PMNs with ICGND, and culture was positive for *N. gonorrhoeae*.

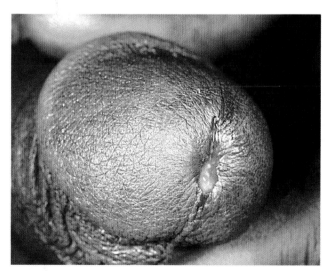

4–6. Mucopurulent exudate in gonorrhea. Some cases lack overtly purulent discharge, and laboratory testing is required to confidently distinguish gonococcal urethritis from NGU.

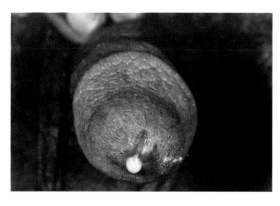

4–7. Copious purulent urethral exudate in gonorrhea.

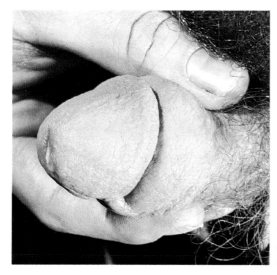

4–8. Gonococcal urethritis with penile venereal edema. When associated with gonorrhea, such edema has been called "bull-headed clap." Penile venereal edema can also occur with genital herpes and chlamydial NGU.

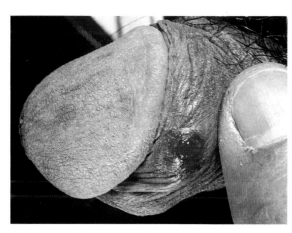

4–9. Presumptive gonococcal ulcer of the penis in a patient with gonococcal urethritis; *N. gonorrhoeae* was isolated from the ulcer as well as the urethra; darkfield microscopy, syphilis serology, and cultures for HSV and *Haemophilus ducreyi* were negative. *N. gonorrhoeae* is a rare cause of ulceration of the genitals or fingers; most cases probably represent secondary gonococcal infection of preexisting skin lesions.

SUGGESTED READING

Bignell C. 2009 European (IUSTI/WHO) guideline on the diagnosis and treatment of gonorrhoea in adults. *Int J STD AIDS.* 2009;20:453-7. *Recommendation of the International Union against STI and the World Health Organization for diagnosis and therapy of gonorrhea in Europe, broadly applicable to most geographic areas.*

Hook EW III, Handsfield HH. Gonococcal infections in the adult. Chapter 35 in KK Holmes, et al., eds. *Sexually Transmitted Diseases.* 4th ed. New York, NY: McGraw-Hill; 2008:627-45. *A comprehensive, state-of-the-art review.*

Hosenfeld CB, et al. Repeat infection with chlamydia and gonorrhea among females: a systematic review of the literature. *Sex Transm Dis.* 2009;36:478-89. *This analysis documents the high priority for rescreening women 3-6 months after treatment for gonorrhea or chlamydia.*

Marcus JL, et al. Sentinel surveillance of rectal chlamydia and gonorrhea among males—San Francisco 2005-2008. *Sex Transm Dis.* 2010;37:59-61. *Documentation of the importance of rectal testing for gonorrhea and chlamydia in evaluating MSM for STD.*

Rice PA. Gonococcal arthritis (disseminated gonococcal infection). *Infect Dis Clin North Am.* 2005;19:853-61. *The most recent comprehensive review of DGI, by one of the leading experts.*

Springer YP, et al. Socioeconomic gradients in sexually transmitted diseases: a geographic information system-based analysis of poverty, race/ethnicity, and gonorrhea rates in California, 2004-2006. *Am J Pub Health.* 2010;100:1060-7. *A sophisticated analysis of demographic and sociological determinants of gonorrhea.*

Tapsall JW. *Neisseria gonorrhoeae* and emerging resistance to extended spectrum cephalosporins. *Curr Opin Infect Dis.* 2009;22:87-91. *A review of trends in emergent gonococcal antibiotic resistance and a warning about the future of treatment with oral cephalosporins.*

5

Syphilis

Syphilis has been recognized as a distinct disorder since the late fifteenth century. It is one of the five originally recognized venereal diseases, along with gonorrhea, lymphogranuloma venereum, chancroid, and donovanosis (granuloma inguinale). Syphilis is characterized by a complex natural history that is largely determined by the unique character of the causative spirochete, *Treponema pallidum*, and the immunologic response to it. The pathogenesis is similar to that of tuberculosis. Both infections are caused by intracellular, slowly replicating pathogens whose containment depends on cell-mediated immunity; both are characterized by an outwardly benign primary infection that is accompanied by silent bacteremia with dissemination of organisms to various organs and by destructive granulomatous inflammation results if infection reactivates, often many years later, due to failure of immune surveillance or overt immunodeficiency.

Syphilis has overlapping primary, secondary, and tertiary stages over several years or decades, interspersed by periods of inactive (latent) infection. Globally, the most serious impact of the disease is from congenital infection, but the most common serious manifestation in adults is neurosyphilis. Although often considered a manifestation of tertiary infection years or decades after acquisition, both subclinical and overt neurological involvement are most common in syphilis under a year in duration. HIV-infected persons with syphilis may have aberrant results of serological tests for syphilis, blunted responses to antibiotic therapy, and perhaps an increased risk of neurosyphilis, but these effects appear to be uncommon. In this respect, the course of syphilis in persons with AIDS is substantially different than that of tuberculosis, despite the parallels in pathogenesis.

The incidence of infectious syphilis (primary, secondary, and early latent infection under a year in duration) fluctuated widely in the United States and Europe throughout the twentieth century, owing to increased case recognition, reporting, and perhaps truly rising incidence in the first half of the century, followed in the second half by rising and falling rates as various risk groups emerged and exhibited great variability in frequency of risk behaviors. Most dramatically in the past 25 years, rates of syphilis in industrialized countries have been driven largely by shifts in sexual behavior among men who have sex with men (MSM) in response to the spread of HIV and by improved treatment and survival in persons with AIDS. By the mid 1990s, the incidence of syphilis in the United States and many industrialized countries had declined to the lowest level at any time since national statistics were complied, and in 1999 the Centers for Disease Control and Prevention (CDC) announced plans to eliminate syphilis in the United States. In many geographic areas, however, a remarkable resurgence began around 2000 and has continued through the present time, with more than a doubling of reported cases through 2009, especially among MSM, many of whom were also infected with HIV.

In addition to MSM, syphilis rates worldwide are highest in the most disadvantaged populations. Population-level herd immunity has been proposed as a partial explanation for varying syphilis rates, but most experts believe the variations are due exclusively to behavioral explanations and societal influences on behavior and access to health care. More than any other STD, except perhaps HIV/AIDS, syphilis thrives in settings of anonymous or furtive sexuality and where economic and social conditions, including poor access to health care, are most problematic. In the United States, heterosexually transmitted syphilis continues at high rates in disadvantaged minority populations, especially in the southeast and along the United States-Mexico border, where congenital syphilis continues to occur at unacceptable rates. Owing to these trends, syphilis elimination in the United States remains a forlorn hope for the foreseeable future. International efforts to control syphilis are largely driven by continued high rates of congenital infection in many developing countries.

EPIDEMIOLOGY

Incidence

- In the United States, 13,997 cases of primary and secondary (P&S) syphilis were reported in 2009; including early latent cases (<1 year duration), incidence in the United States approximates 31,000 cases annually

- Reported incidence of P&S syphilis rose 119% from 2000 (2.1 cases per 100,000) to 2009 (4.6 per 100,000)

- Geographic variability is great; 70% of U.S. counties reported no cases in 2009

- European Union had 17,603 reported cases (all stages) in 2007 (4.4 per 100,000); most countries had rates ranging from 1 to 8 per 100,000; in many countries, recently rising rates in MSM parallel U.S. trend

- Highest rates are in southern Africa and parts of Asia

Transmission

- Sexually transmissible only during primary, secondary, and early latent stages

- Requires exposure to moist mucocutaneous lesions (chancre, mucous patches, condylomata lata) that teem with spirochetes

- Congenital syphilis results from transplacental infection

- Rare cases of nonsexual transmission, typically from direct contact with infected persons' nongenital lesions (e.g., nursing, premastication of infant food in some cultures)

Age

- All ages are susceptible

- Peak rates occur at older ages than most STDs; in the United States, 57% of reported P&S cases in 2009 were ≥30 years old (vs. 12% of chlamydia and 20% of gonorrhea cases)

- Late syphilis often diagnosed in persons ≥50 years of age

Sex and Sexual Orientation

- Both sexes equally susceptible

- Population level sex distribution largely reflects proportion of cases in MSM; male:female ratio of reported P&S syphilis rose from 1.2 to 1 in 1996 to 5-6 to 1 from 2007 to 2009; trends are similar in many industrialized countries, especially in western Europe

- In King County, Washington 2009 annual rate of early syphilis estimated 342 per 100,000 MSM and 1,169 cases per 100,000 HIV-infected MSM (vs. 0.4 per 100,000 heterosexual men)

- High rates in HIV-infected MSM may be attributed in part to selection of partners of like HIV status (serosorting)

- Rare in exclusively homosexual women

Race/Ethnicity

- Race and ethnicity are markers of socioeconomic status, access to health care, education, and sexual network patterns (Chap. 1)

- Reported rates of P&S syphilis, the United States, 2009
  - Whites 4,256 cases (2.1 per 100,000)
  - African Americans 7,335 cases (19.2 per 100,000)
  - Hispanics 2,112 cases (4.5 per 100,000)
  - Asian/Pacific Island ancestry 225 cases (1.6 per 100,000)
  - Native Americans 61 cases (2.4 per 100,000)

Other Risk Factors

- Anonymous sexual partnerships

- Illicit drug use

- Commercial or coerced sex

- Low socioeconomic and educational attainment

- Population migration

- War and other settings of social disruption

- Undocumented immigrants in the United States

CLINICAL MANIFESTATIONS

Epidemiologic and Exposure History

- Almost all persons with infectious syphilis acknowledge new sex partner or a partner who has other sexual relationships

- Unprotected sex, especially with anonymous or commercial partners

- Among males, sex with other men

- Heterosexual men and women affected by societal conditions addressed above

Symptoms and Examination

Primary Syphilis

- Incubation period 2–6 weeks, occasionally up to 3 months, from exposure to clinically evident primary syphilis

- Chancre often presents as a single painless or minimally painful round or oval ulcer, typically indurated, with a "clean" base with little or no purulent exudate

- Presence of classic chancre is insensitive but highly specific for diagnosis of syphilis; i.e. many chancres lack classic appearance, but most typical chancres are syphilitic

- Location: primarily sites most exposed during sexual activity

  ○ External genitals (penile head and shaft, labia minor, vaginal introitus)

  ○ Intravaginal or anal lesions also are common

  ○ Oral chancres occur occasionally, depending on sexual practices

- Regional lymphadenopathy is common, generally bilateral, with firm, nonfluctuant, nontender or mildly tender nodes, without overlying erythema

- No systemic symptoms

- Asymptomatic infection is common, primarily due to chancres hidden from view (e.g., vaginal, anal, oral, or rectal)

- All clinical manifestations and course may be highly variable; atypical presentations are common

Secondary Syphilis

- May overlap with primary, e.g. persistent chancre in patients with secondary manifestations

- Most common presentation is generalized papulosquamous, nonpruritic skin rash, often involving palms and soles

- Atypical rashes, including pruritic ones, may occur

- Protean manifestations (syphilis has been called "the great imitator"): mucous patches (painless mucous membrane lesions), condylomata lata (genital or perianal warty excrescences), patchy ("moth-eaten") alopecia, generalized lymphadenopathy, hepatosplenomegaly, abdominal pain due to gastric ulceration, fever, malaise, headache, immune complex polyarthritis, others

Neurosyphilis

- Early neurosyphilis occurs during secondary and early latent infection

- Main clinical manifestations of early neurosyphilis reflect meningovascular involvement: cranial nerve palsies, headache, hearing loss, vestibular dysfunction (e.g., vertigo), arterial occlusion (typically involving mid-size arteries) resulting in stroke

- Iritis and uveitis are common; syphilitic ocular disease always implies neurosyphilis and requires similar management

Tertiary (Late) Syphilis

- Classic tertiary syphilis now rare in most of the world; almost unheard of in the United States and western Europe, perhaps because many persons with latent syphilis receive incidental antibiotic therapy

- Main features are locally destructive granulomatous lesions (gummas) of skin, liver, bones, or other organs
- Signs of late neurosyphilis include tabes dorsalis and dementia, often with paranoid features ("general paresis")
- Cardiovascular manifestations, e.g. ascending aortic aneurysm and aortic valve insufficiency, are now rare

Latent Syphilis

- By definition, asymptomatic infection at any time following primary syphilis
- Only detectable serologically
- Early latent (≤1 year, infectious) and late latent (>1 year, usually not transmissible)
- The distinction between early and late latent syphilis often is moot because duration is difficult to determine

Congenital Syphilis

- Severity ranges from asymptomatic to fatal
- Common early manifestations are spontaneous abortion, stillbirth, encephalitis, generalized skin rash, rhinitis ("snuffles"), hepatic dysfunction, consumption coagulopathy, multiple organ failure
- Later manifestations, usually not apparent at birth, include osteitis of long bones, maxillofacial and dental malformations, keratitis, neurosensory hearing loss, and chronic neuropsychological deficits

LABORATORY DIAGNOSIS

Identification of *T. pallidum*

- *T. pallidum* cannot be grown *in vitro*; no culture test exists
- Detection depends on visual, antigenic, or genetic detection
- Visualization requires darkfield or phase microscopy, or special staining techniques (e.g., silver stain, immunofluorescence)

Darkfield Microscopy

- Suitable specimens include saline-mounted scrapings from chancre or mucocutaneous lesion of secondary syphilis, or lymph node aspirate
- Identification of motile spirochetes typical of *T. pallidum*: 10–13 μm in length, one spiral turn per μm, characteristic rotational motility and flexion
- Performance of darkfield microscopy is poor for oral and anorectal lesions owing to frequent commensal spiral organisms with appearance similar to *T. pallidum*

Immunologic and Genetic Detection

- Polyclonal fluorescent antibody test is a specific and moderately sensitive substitute for darkfield microscopy, but not widely avaialable
- Sensitive and specific fluorescent mononclonal antibody and polymerase chain reaction (PCR) assays have been developed, but to date not commercially available

Histopathology

- Silver stain or immunofluorescence microscopy of infected tissues

- Insensitive but specific, sometimes diagnostic

Serology

- Serological antibody tests are the mainstay of laboratory diagnosis for all stages of syphilis other than primary

Nontreponemal Tests

- Venereal Disease Research Laboratory (VDRL) test and variants, including rapid plasma reagin (RPR) and toluidine red unheated serum reagin test (TRUST)

- Descendents of the earliest serological tests (e.g., Wassermann)

- Detect antibody to cardiolipin (diphosphatidylchonine), a component of normal mammalian cell membranes and incorporated into *T. pallidum*

- Sensitive for all stages except primary syphilis

- Nonspecific; positive results require confirmation with a treponemal test

- Titer varies with activity of infection; useful to assess therapeutic response

Treponemal Antibody Tests

- Antibody to *T. pallidum*-specific antigens

- Agglutination tests, e.g. *T. pallidum* particle agglutination (TPPA), *T. pallidum* hemagglutination (TPHA), and microhemagglutination assay for *T. pallidum* (MHA-TP)

- Fluorescent treponemal antibody-absorbed (FTA-ABS) is historic gold standard; labor-intensive and now infrequently employed, but remains useful when other tests give uncertain results

- Enzyme immunoassay (EIA), easily automated and suitable for efficient testing of large numbers of specimens; now widely available and increasingly used for screening

- Rapid assays using fluid flow technologies (e.g., dipstick); not yet commercially available in the United States

Use and Interpretation of Serological Tests

For most of the twentieth century, initial diagnostic testing and serological screening were undertaken with a nontreponemal assay such as VDRL, RPR, or TRUST. Newly positive results with these tests require confirmation with a *T. pallidum*-specific antibody test such as MHA-TP, TPPA, or FTA-ABS. However, in recent years the development and rapid adoption of low-cost, high-throughput *T. pallidum*-specific tests using EIA and other technologies, and rapid dipstick testing in some settings, have led to use of treponemal assays for screening and initial diagnostic testing. RPR, VDRL, and TRUST retain their historic advantage of easy quantitation by dilutional titer, required for clinical staging and to monitor the response to therapy. Thus, the historic testing sequence often is now reversed: a *T. pallidum*-specific test such as EIA is performed first, followed by quantitative VDRL, RPR, or TRUST to assess disease activity. Regardless of testing sequence, persons with newly positive results on either type of test typically require repeat testing with the alternate method.

The nontreponemal tests become reactive during primary syphilis, and about 70% of persons with primary syphilis have positive results. The nontreponemal titer peaks in the secondary stage, usually at a titer of 1:16 to 1:256, and declines thereafter, typically falling to 1:4 or lower in untreated late-latent infection. The titer usually rises again if there is progression to tertiary syphilis, although exceptions are frequent and some patients with tertiary disease have low titers. Nontreponemal reactivity declines in response to successful treatment. For successfully treated primary and secondary syphilis, the titer declines by at least 2 dilutions (e.g., from 1:16 to 1:4, or from 1:64 to 1:16 or lower) within 3 months, and in 90% of patients the VDRL/RPR becomes negative by 12 months. In late syphilis, by contrast, low titers (usually 1:1–1:4) may persist after successful treatment. VDRL and RPR titers often vary from one another by one or two dilutions, and it is important that the same test, preferably performed in the same laboratory, be used to follow the serological response to treatment.

Biological false-positive results (i.e., reactive VDRL, RPR, or TRUST with negative treponemal test results) occasionally occur, often associated with pregnancy or immunologic disorders; the titer usually is 1:8 or lower. Classical biological false-positive results probably will become less common as *T. pallidum*-specific EIAs or other tests are used for initial screening; with negative results, nontreponemal testing will not be performed.

The treponemal tests FTA-ABS, MHA-TP, and TPPA revert to negative in up to 25% of persons treated for primary syphilis, but they remain positive indefinitely when treatment is delayed to the secondary stage or later. Once a treponemal antibody test is positive, repeat testing rarely is indicated; only the quantitative nontreponemal tests are used to monitor disease activity. Beyond the primary stage, active syphilis is rare if the VDRL or RPR test is negative. However, the duration and durability of seropositivity by EIA and other newer treponemal antibody tests have not been rigorously studied. Therefore, the clinical status, prognosis, and need for treatment are unknown among persons screened for syphilis and found to have reactive EIA but negative VDRL, RPR, or TRUST, especially in those seemingly at lifelong low risk for syphilis. Many such patients also have negative results with MHA-TP, TPPA, and FTA-ABS, creating diagnostic and therapeutic dilemmas, especially in persons seemingly at low risk for syphilis. Research to resolve these uncertainties is a high priority.

Cerebrospinal Fluid Examination

Neurosyphilis is the most common complication of syphilis and occurs primarily during early syphilis <1 year in duration. Examination of cerebrospinal fluid (CSF), obtained by lumbar puncture, is the primary diagnostic tool. No "gold standard" for CSF diagnosis of neurosyphilis exists. Reactive CSF–VDRL is highly specific and considered proof of neurosyphilis, but is insensitive, missing a substantial proportion of cases. Elevated CSF mononuclear leukocytes or CSF protein are strong indicators of probable neurosyphilis in patients with positive blood tests for syphilis. *T. pallidum*-specific serological tests on CSF (e.g., TPPA or FTA-ABS) are believed to be nonspecific and do not confirm a diagnosis of neurosyphilis. Clinicians evaluating patients for neurosyphilis are encouraged to consult with an expert.

The primary indications for CSF examination are neurological symptoms or signs in persons with syphilis of any stage or duration. CSF examination also is indicated for patients whose VDRL or RPR titer does not decline at least 2 dilutions after treatment of syphilis, because low-dose penicillin (i.e., benzathine penicillin) may not eradicate *T. pallidum* sequestered in the central nervous system. For patients with syphilis >1 year in duration, without neurological symptoms, indications for CSF examination are VDRL or RPR titer ≥1:32; HIV infection; other signs or symptoms of active syphilis; or planned treatment with an antibiotic other than penicillin. Whether CSF examination should be routine in some patients with syphilis <1 year in duration, absent neurological symptoms or signs—i.e., to detect sub-clinical neurosyphilis and provide enhanced therapy, especially in HIV-infected patients—is a matter of current debate.

TREATMENT

Principles Antibiotic levels sufficient to inhibit *T. pallidum* should be maintained in blood and infected tissues for at least 10 days for early syphilis and 4 weeks for late syphilis. The organism remains exquisitely sensitive to penicillin, which is rapidly treponemacidal, and penicillin G remains the drug of choice for all stages of the disease. Other penicillins, such as ampicillin and amoxicillin, are active but require multiple dose daily treatment for prolonged periods, making compliance difficult, and few clinical studies have documented clinical efficacy. Doxycycline and other tetracyclines are somewhat less active against *T. pallidum*, but owing to favorable pharmacokinetics and dosing frequency, they usually are used when penicillin cannot be given. Ceftriaxone is highly active against *T. pallidum* and sometimes is used when penicillin cannot be given, but clinical experience is limited. Azithromycin is an attractive oral treatment alternative that has proved effective against early syphilis in single 2.0 g doses. Unfortunately, the frequency of *T. pallidum* strains resistant to the macrolide antibiotics, once rare, is rising in some geographic areas, including parts of North America and Europe. Azithromycin may be useful in selected settings where resistance has not yet emerged, but all macrolides should be used with great caution, if at all, in most clinical settings. Most other antibiotic classes, including the fluoroquinolones, sulfonamides, and aminoglycosides, have no antitreponemal activity.

Many patients with early syphilis and a few with late syphilis experience Jarisch-Herxheimer reactions soon after onset of treatment, with fever, chills, malaise, headache, and sometimes increased prominence of the chancre, skin rash, or lymphadenopathy. The reaction is believed to result from release of treponemal antigens following rapid killing of *T. pallidum*; it typically begins 6–12 hours after treatment and resolves within 24 hours. Nonsteroidal anti-inflammatory drugs such as ibuprofen may speed symptomatic relief.

Recommended Regimens
Primary, Secondary, and Early Latent Infection
Treatment of Choice

- Benzathine penicillin G 2.4 million units IM, single dose

Alternative Regimens for Penicillin-allergic Patients

- Doxycycline 100 mg PO *bid* for 2 weeks
- Tetracycline HCl 500 mg PO *qid* for 2 weeks
- Alternative regimens should be avoided for HIV-infected patients; those allergic to penicillin should be desensitized and treated with penicillin

Late Syphilis (>1 Year Duration), Except Neurosyphilis
Treatment of Choice

- Benzathine penicillin G 2.4 million units IM once weekly for 3 doses

Alternative Regimens

- Doxycycline 100 mg orally *bid* for 4 weeks
- Tetracycline HCl 500 mg orally *qid* for 4 weeks

Neurosyphilis

Treatment of Choice

- Aqueous penicillin G 3–4 million units IV every 4 hours for 10 to 14 days

Alternative Regimen

- Procaine penicillin G 2.4 million units IM once daily, plus probenecid 500 mg PO *qid*, for 10–14 days
- Only penicillin is known to be effective; penicillin-allergic patients should be desensitized and treated with penicillin

Syphilis in Pregnant Women

- Treat with penicillin, appropriate to clinical stage
- Allergic patients should be desensitized and treated with penicillin
- Tetracyclines are contraindicated in pregnancy and erythromycin does not treat fetal infection

Congenital Syphilis

- Treatment issues are complex
- Treat with penicillin in consultation with an expert

Follow-up

Primary, Secondary, and Early Latent Syphilis

- Reexamine and obtain quantitative VDRL, RPR, or TRUST 1, 3, 6, and 12 months after treatment or until negative
- If VDRL, RPR, or TRUST remains reactive at any titer, repeat at 6- to 12-month intervals for 1–2 years

Late Syphilis

- Reexamine and obtain quantitative VDRL, RPR, or TRUST after 3, 6, and 12 months
- If test remains reactive at 12 months, repeat at 12-month intervals for 2–3 years

HIV-infected Patients

- Reexamine and obtain quantitative VDRL, RPR, or TRUST 1, 2, 3, 6, 9, 12, and 24 months after treatment, even if test becomes negative before 24 months

Neurosyphilis

- Follow as appropriate for stage and HIV status
- If CSF abnormal before treatment, repeat CSF examination at 6-month intervals until cell count is within normal limits and CSF–VDRL negative

Management of Sex Partners

- Examine and obtain serologic tests for syphilis for all sex partners exposed during infectious period, usually from exposure to start of treatment

- Treat seronegative partners who have had sex with an infectious case within preceding 3 months, using benzathine penicillin or other regimen effective against early syphilis
- In the United States and western Europe, local or regional health authorities usually will assist in identifying and notifying partners

PREVENTION

Screening

- Routine serology for persons at risk, especially those with characteristics of core transmitters
- Most states and many countries' public health authorities recommend or require testing of all pregnant women

Reporting

- Required by law in all states in the United States and regional health authorities in most industrialized countries
- Reporting and epidemiologic analysis are instrumental to allocate resources, target prevention programs, and facilitate counseling and partner management services

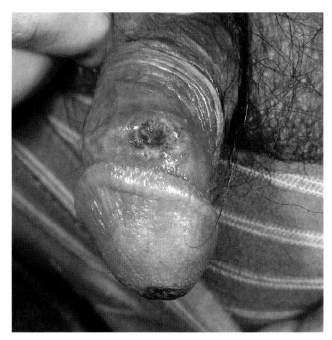

5–1. Chancre of penis in primary syphilis.

CASE

Patient Profile Age 25, MSM, computer programmer

History Painless sore on penis for 10 days; frequently has sex with anonymous partners; "usually" uses condoms for anal but not oral sex; negative test for HIV 3 months earlier

Examination Indurated, nontender ulcer of penis, without purulent exudate; bilateral inguinal lymphadenopathy with 2- to 3-cm rubbery, slightly tender nodes

Differential Diagnosis Classic chancre is highly specific for syphilis, but consider herpes and chancroid; slim possibility of cancer, pyogenic infection, and other nonsexually transmitted conditions

Laboratory Darkfield microscopy positive for *T. pallidum*; stat RPR positive; VDRL positive (titer 1:8), TPPA reactive; lesion culture for herpes simplex virus (negative); rectal NAATs for *N. gonorrhoeae* and *C. trachomatis*, pharyngeal culture for *N. gonorrhoeae* (all negative); HIV serology (negative)

Diagnosis Primary syphilis

Treatment Benzathine penicillin G 2.4 million units IM

Management of Partners Patient interviewed by health department counselor; no identifiable partners

Comment Classic presentation of primary syphilis; treatment would have been warranted even if darkfield and serological tests for syphilis had been negative; patient counseled about HIV risks and prevention; follow-up syphilis serology scheduled after 1, 3, 6, and 12 months

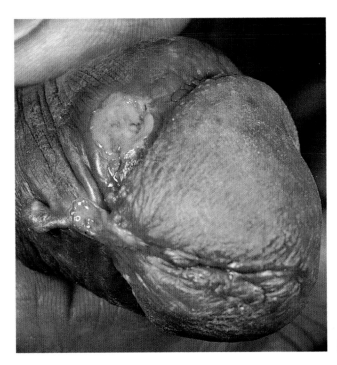

5–2. Two penile chancres in primary syphilis.

CASE

Patient Profile Age 32, married assembly line worker with 4-year history of recurrent genital herpes

History Two penile sores 3 weeks; "I thought my herpes was back"; treated 5 years previously for secondary syphilis; occasional anonymous sex with other men in bars or parks

Examination Two indurated, slightly tender penile lesions, with firmly adherent white exudate; bilateral, shotty, nontender inguinal lymphadenopathy

Differential Diagnosis Primary syphilis, recurrent herpes, possible chancroid

Laboratory Darkfield examination positive for spirochetes; stat RPR positive; VDRL reactive, titer 1:64; HSV culture negative; HIV serology negative

Diagnosis Primary syphilis

Treatment Benzathine penicillin G 2.4 million units IM

Management of Partners Patient referred his wife, in whom VDRL was negative; treated with benzathine penicillin G

Other Presentation with two lesions, past history of genital herpes, and the purulent-appearing exudate suggested possibility of genital herpes, but herpes rarely persists for >2 weeks, and multiple chancres occasionally occur in syphilis. A confirmatory treponemal antibody test (e.g., TPPA) was not done, because positive results would be expected due to prior secondary syphilis. The patient was scheduled for repeat HIV serology after 3 months and, at his request, was referred for professional counseling to address his compulsive risky sexual behavior.

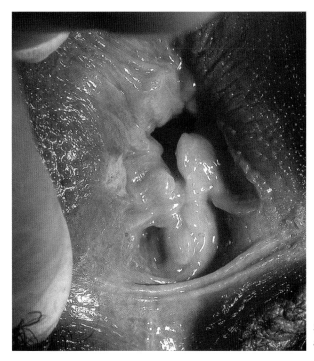

5–3. Primary syphilis: darkfield-positive chancre; atypically tender, nonindurated lesion.

CASE

Patient Profile Age 22, unemployed, crack cocaine addict; denied commercial sex but in past years "sometimes" accepted money or drugs from partners

History Painful genital sore for 5 days; only recent sex partner was her boyfriend, who also used cocaine

Examination Superficial, tender ulcer of vestibule; no lymphadenopathy or skin rash

Differential Diagnosis Genital herpes, chancroid, syphilis, trauma; less likely considerations included Behçet disease, Stevens-Johnson syndrome, and others

Laboratory Darkfield microscopy positive for *T. pallidum*; stat RPR (negative); lesion culture for HSV (negative); cervical cultures for *N. gonorrhoeae* and *C. trachomatis* (both negative); HIV serology negative

Diagnosis Primary syphilis

Treatment Benzathine penicillin G 2.4 million units IM

Partner Management Partner was referred and found to have latent syphilis of unknown duration, with VDRL tier 1:16 and reactive TPPA; treated with benzathine penicillin G

Comment The clinical presentation suggested herpes or chancroid, based on the painful, tender, non-indurated genital ulcer, illustrating the nonspecific nature of some chancres. Up to 40% of patients with primary syphilis present before developing reactive serological tests, especially if tested within 2 weeks of onset. The patient was advised to return for follow-up syphilis serology testing after 1, 3, 6, and 12 months.

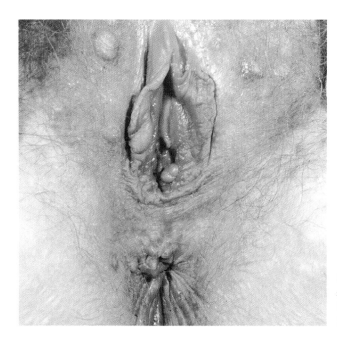

5–4. Condylomata lata in secondary syphilis; such lesions contain large numbers of *T. pallidum* (often darkfield-positive) and are highly infectious.

CASE

Patient Profile Age 19, single beautician

History Referred for consultation because of genital and perianal warts of 6 weeks' duration, not responding to weekly applications of podophyllin; 3 sex partners in previous 6 months; unconfirmed history of "severe reaction" to penicillin in early childhood

Examination Several flat, firm, slightly erythematous papular excrescences of perineum and perinatally; some perianal lesions superficially ulcerated; bilateral nontender inguinal lymphadenopathy; oral examination and skin of scalp, trunk, and extremities normal

Differential Diagnosis Secondary syphilis, genital warts, herpes

Laboratory Darkfield microscopy negative; stat RPR positive; VDRL positive, titer 1:128; TPPA positive; HIV serology, PCR for HSV, NAATs for *C. trachomatis* and *N. gonorrhoeae* (all negative)

Diagnosis Secondary syphilis with condylomata lata

Treatment Doxycycline 100 mg PO *bid* for 2 weeks

Partner Management Two of the patient's 3 recent sex partners located and treated; one had latent syphilis of unknown duration and the other was uninfected; third was not located

Comment The diagnosis was delayed because syphilis serology was not done because the referring clinician believed the patient had genital warts due to HPV. Doxycycline was prescribed because of history of penicillin allergy. All lesions resolved within 1 week. Follow-up syphilis serology was scheduled at 1, 3, 6, and 12 months.

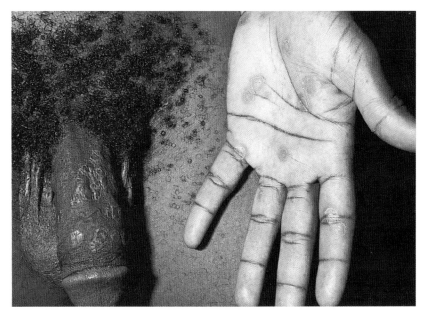

5–5. Secondary syphilis rash of penis and palms.

CASE

Patient Profile Age 36, unemployed, IV drug user

History Painless, nonpruritic rash of hands, trunk, and penis for 3 months; anorexia with 10-lb weight loss; recalled a penile sore "a few months ago" that went away; "several" female sex partners in past year

Examination Slim, ill-appearing; papulosquamous eruption of trunk, genitals, extremities, palms, and soles; generalized nontender lymphadenopathy (cervical, inguinal, supraclavicular)

Differential Diagnosis Secondary syphilis, pityriasis rosea, viral syndrome, allergic rash, HIV infection

Laboratory Stat RPR positive; VDRL reactive, titer 1:512; TPPA positive; HIV serology positive; HIV viral load 1.2 million, CD4 lymphocyte count 320 cells per mm^3; underwent lumbar puncture for CSF examination: cells and protein normal, CSF–VDRL negative

Diagnosis Secondary syphilis; HIV infection

Treatment Benzathine penicillin G 2.4 million units IM, single dose

Partner Management Patient cooperated with health department counselor to identify, locate, and treat three sex and/or needle-sharing partners; one had latent syphilis, unknown duration (VDRL titer 1:4); all were HIV negative

Comment The rash cleared promptly after penicillin therapy, but lymphadenopathy persisted and was judged as resulting from HIV rather than syphilis. CSF examination was undertaken in light of recommendations by some experts that asymptomatic neurosyphilis be excluded in HIV-infected patients with nontreponemal antibody titer ≥1:32 and CD4 count <350 cells per mm^3. Follow-up syphilis serology at 1, 2, 3, 6, 9, 12, and 24 months.

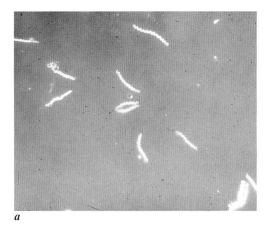 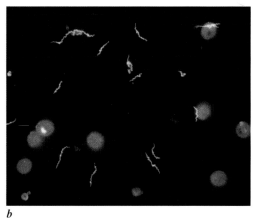

a *b*

5–6. *Treponema pallidum. a.* Viewed by darkfield microscopy. *b.* Stained with fluorescein-conjugated monoclonal antibody to *T. pallidum*, with Evans Blue counterstain, viewed by fluorescence microscopy. (*Courtesy of Sheila A. Lukehart, Ph.D.*)

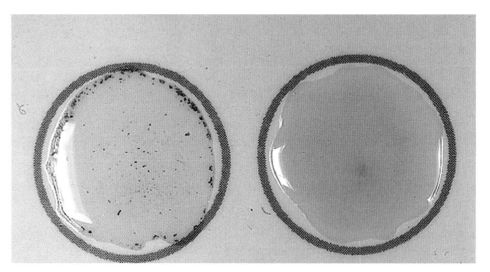

5–7. Rapid plasma reagin (RPR) card test. Reactive serum (left) shows agglutination of carbon particles; control specimen (right) shows no agglutination. The RPR card test requires 10 minutes to perform. (Enlarged view; circles on RPR card are 1.5 cm in diameter.)

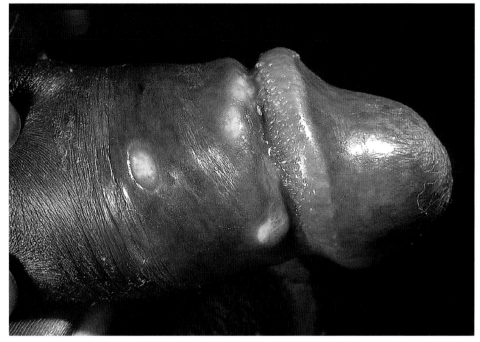

5–8. Primary syphilis: multiple chancres of the penis, under the retracted foreskin. Multiple chancres occasionally occur, perhaps with increased frequency in moist areas such as the preputial sac. Pearly penile papules also are present on the corona.

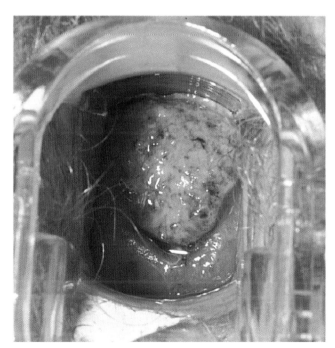

5–9. Primary syphilis: atypical hypertrophic chancre of cervix. The patient presented with a complaint of postcoital bleeding and was initially thought to have cervical carcinoma, but syphilis was confirmed by dark-field examination, serology, and rapid resolution of the lesion following benzathine penicillin G.

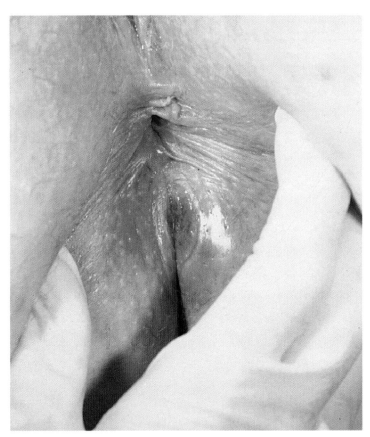

5–10. Primary syphilis: darkfield-positive perianal chancre, atypically nonindurated.

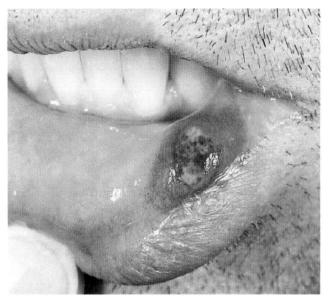

5–11. Primary syphilis: chancre of lower lip. Although less common than genital or perianal lesions, oral chancres are not rare.

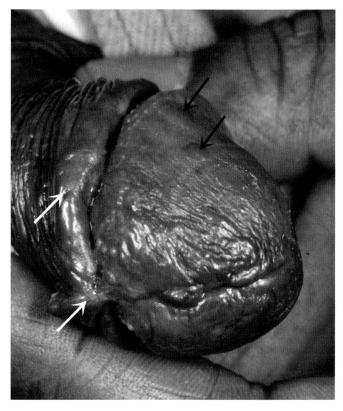

5-12. Primary and secondary syphilis in a man with AIDS, showing two darkfield-positive chancres (white arrows) and papular lesions of secondary syphilis (black arrows). The patient also had a generalized maculopapular rash consistent with secondary syphilis and VDRL was reactive at a titer of 1:64. Anecdotal reports suggest that progression from primary to secondary syphilis sometimes may be accelerated in HIV-infected patients.

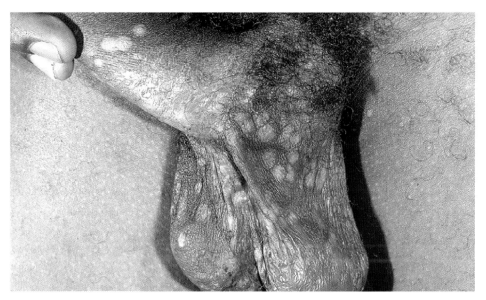

5–13. Secondary syphilis: papular eruption of penis and scrotum. Depigmented lesions are common in dark-skinned persons.

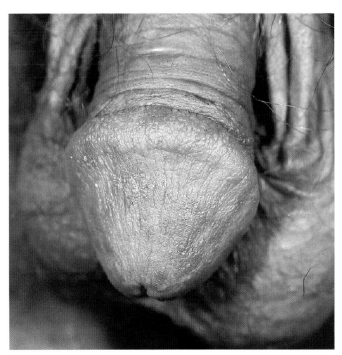

5–14. Secondary syphilis: papulosquamous rash of penis. Note similarity to scabies (see Fig. 14–2) and psoriasis (see Figs. 22–5 and 22–6).

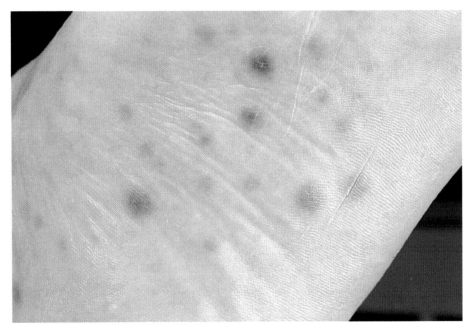

5–15. Secondary syphilis: papular rash of the sole of the foot.

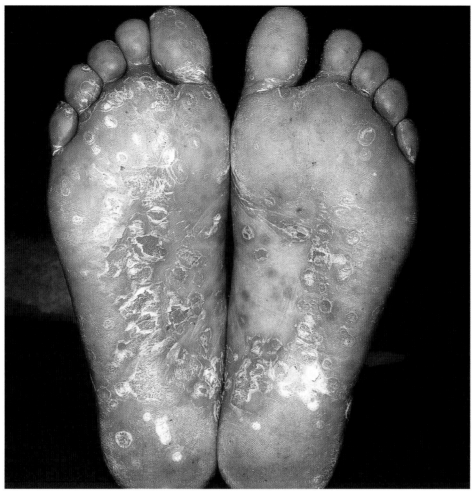

5–16. Secondary syphilis: extensive hyperkeratotic plantar rash in an HIV-infected man with secondary syphilis. Note similarity to keratoderma blennorrhagica of reactive arthritis (see Fig. 17–3).

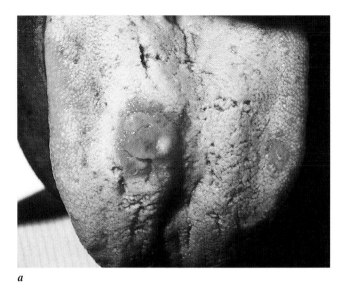

a

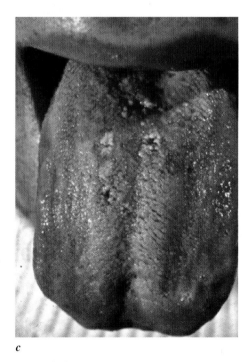

b

c

5-17. Lesions of the tongue in secondary syphilis. *a.* Mucous patch. *b.* Multiple mucous patches. *c.* Mucous patches and ulcerations. Mucous patches are superficial ulcerations of mucous membrane and other moist surfaces, teeming with spirochetes and highly infectious, probably accounting for many transmissions by persons with apparently asymptomatic syphilis.

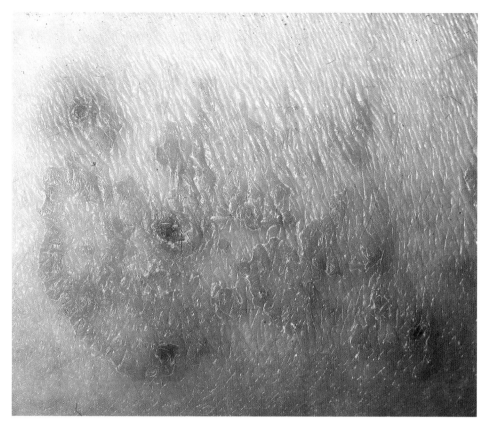

5–18. Secondary syphilis: atypical eczema-like rash of buttock. Despite its dry appearance, this lesion was darkfield-positive and resolved promptly after treatment with benzathine penicillin G.

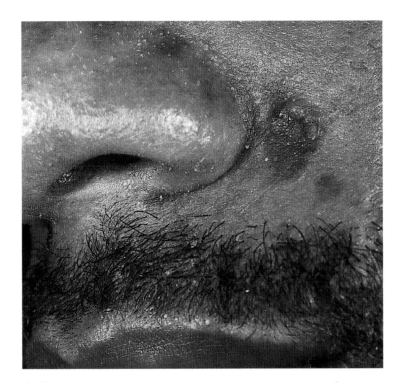

5–19. Secondary syphilis: hyperpigmented papules of the nose and nasolabial fold.

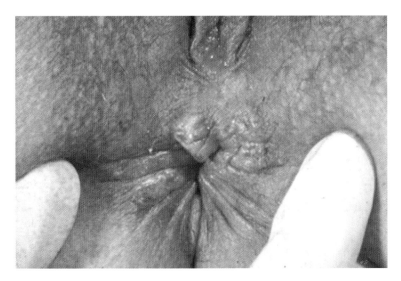

5–20. Secondary syphilis: superficially ulcerated condylomata lata of the anus.

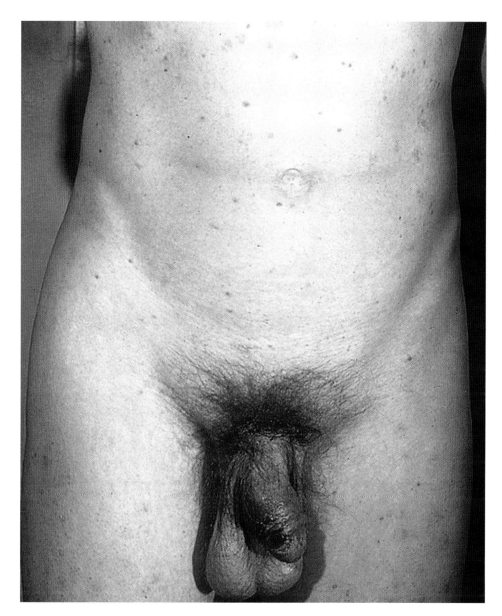

5–21. Secondary syphilis: papulosquamous rash involving trunk and extremities. This HIV-infected patient also had a large necrotic penile ulcer with streptococcal cellulitis, possibly the result of secondary infection of the original chancre. Before the penile infection supervened, the patient's physician was unaware that the patient continued to be sexually active with multiple anonymous partners, and the physician failed to perform a syphilis serology, believing the rash was due to allergy to antiretroviral drugs. This is the same patient whose penile lesion is illustrated in Fig. 22–16.

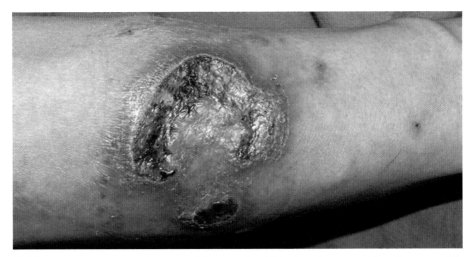

5–22. Extensive cutaneous ulceration of the arm of an HIV-infected patient with malignant syphilis (lues maligna). A rare complication of early syphilis, malignant syphilis has clinical characteristics similar to those of gummas associated with tertiary syphilis. Recent case reports suggest that malignant syphilis may be relatively frequent in HIV-infected persons. (*Courtesy of Dr. Naoki Yanagisawa and Reprinted with permission from Yanagisawa N, Imamura A. Clin Infect Dis. 2008;47:1068-9.*)

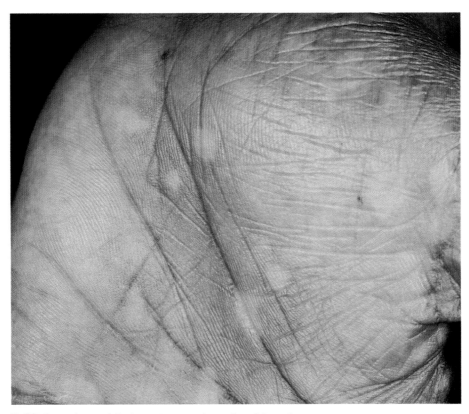

5–23. Secondary syphilis: hypopigmented macules of the palms.

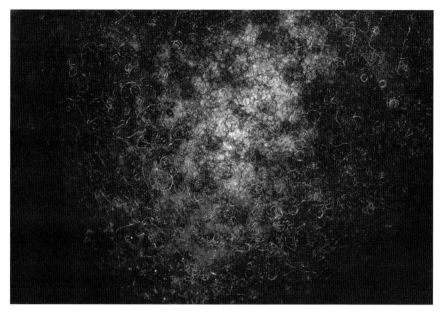

5–24. Patchy ("moth-eaten") alopecia in secondary syphilis. (*Reprinted with permission from Interactive Health Media, LLC.*)

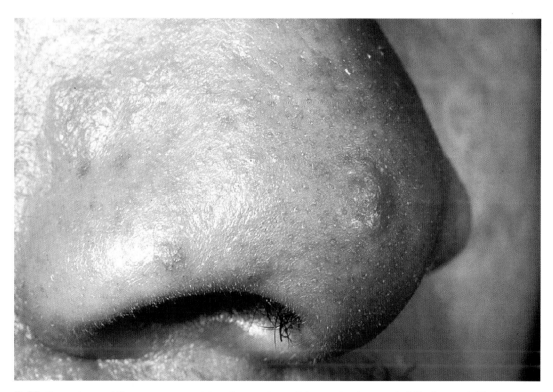

5–25. Secondary syphilis: cutaneous nodules of nose; the nodules resolved promptly following penicillin therapy.

SUGGESTED READING

DiCarlo RP, Martin DH. The clinical diagnosis of genital ulcer disease in men. *Clin Infect Dis.* 1997;25:292-8. *Study of 446 men with genital ulcers, showing that typical chancres are specific for syphilis, but insensitive; and that otherwise ulcer morphology poorly predicts etiology.*

Ghanem KG, et al. Lumbar puncture in HIV-infected patients with syphilis and no neurological symptoms. *Clin Infect Dis.* 2009;48:816-21. *A clinical trial concluding that nontreponemal antibody titer and CD4 count offer improved prediction of neurosyphilis compared with stage-based criteria.*

Hawkes S. Eliminating congenital syphilis: if not now then when? [Editorial] *Sex Transm Dis.* 2009;36:714-20. *An editorial that addresses the global epidemiology and prevention of congenital syphilis.*

Holmes KK. Azithromycin versus penicillin G benzathine for early syphilis [Editorial]. *N Engl J Med.* 2005;353:1291-3. *A warning against routine use of azithromycin for syphilis unless macrolide resistance is excluded.*

Hook EW III, et al. A phase III equivalence trial of azithromycin versus benzathine penicillin for treatment of early syphilis. *J Infect Dis.* 2010;201:1729-35. *A well designed trial demonstrating single-dose azithromycin efficacy comparable to that of benzathine penicillin in geographic areas without demonstrated* T. pallidum *resistance to macrolides.*

Kerani RP, et al. Rising rates of syphilis in the era of syphilis elimination. *Sex Transm Dis.* 2007;34:154-61. *An observational study documenting high and rising rates of syphilis among men who have sex with men in a mid-sized US city.*

Li JZ, et al. Ocular syphilis among HIV-infected individuals. *Clin Infect Dis.* 2010;51:468-71. *Report of 13 cases, some of whom relapsed despite recommended penicillin therapy.*

Mitchell SJ, et al. Azithromycin-resistant syphilis infection: San Francisco, California, 2000-2004. *Clin Infect Dis.* 2005;42:337-45. *Documentation of rapid evolution and spread of macrolide-resistant* T. pallidum, *perhaps in response to use of azithromycin for treatment.*

Seña AC, et al. Novel *Treponema pallidum* serological tests: a paradigm shift in syphilis screening for the 21st century. *Clin Infect Dis.* 2010;51:700-8. *A review of clinical implications and interpretations of* T. pallidum-*specific serological tests for screening and diagnostic testing.*

Sparling PF, et al. Clinical manifestations of syphilis. Chapter 37 in KK Holmes, et al., eds. *Sexually Transmitted Diseases.* 4th ed. New York, NY: McGraw-Hill; 2008:661-84. *An up-to-date review in the primary textbook on STD.*

6

Chancroid

Chancroid is a genital ulcer disease caused by *Haemophilus ducreyi*, and one of the original five venereal diseases, along with gonorrhea, syphilis, lymphogranuloma venereum, and donovanosis. Chancroid was the first STD recognized to enhance the efficiency of sexual transmission of HIV. Although endemic in parts of the world, notably sub-Saharan Africa, Asia, and Latin America, in most areas chancroid is declining in incidence and has largely been supplanted by genital herpes as the most common cause of genital ulcer disease. Chancroid is currently rare in North America and western Europe but has the potential to reappear in localized outbreaks. Recent reports suggest occasional nonsexual transmission in tropical settings, based on identification of *H. ducreyi* in chronic lower leg ulcers of patients in the South Pacific. Autoinoculation lesions can occur in patients with sexually acquired chancroid, supporting the potential for nonsexual transmission. Diagnosis of chancroid is difficult, owing to unreliability of clinical criteria, insensitivity of *H. ducreyi* culture in routine laboratories, and lack of readily available alternative methods. However, it is likely that polymerase chain reaction (PCR) or other sensitive nucleic acid amplification tests will be available in the future.

EPIDEMIOLOGY

Incidence and Prevalence

- Declining incidence in the United States since 1990s; 17–30 reported cases per year 2004–2009
- True frequency may be higher, because of difficulties in recognition and diagnosis, but nevertheless very rare
- Occasional localized outbreaks, usually in socioeconomically disadvantaged populations
- Remains common in some developing countries

Transmission

- Historically, thought to be transmitted exclusively by sexual contact
- Autoinoculation or contamination of preexisting cutaneous ulcers apparently explains some non-genital cases

Age

- All ages susceptible
- Most cases age 25–35 years

Sex

- No known predilection
- Reported cases primarily in men
- Clinical recognition and diagnosis are more difficult in women

Sexual Orientation

- No predilection known

Other Risk Factors

- Being uncircumcised probably elevates risk in men

HISTORY

Incubation Period

- Usually 2–5 days, up to 14 days

Symptoms

- Initial inflammatory papule with rapid progression to painful ulceration (1–2 days)
- Usually single lesions, sometimes multiple
- 50% of patients have painful regional (usually inguinal) lymphadenopathy
- No systemic symptoms
- Asymptomatic carriage of *H. ducreyi* is controversial, probably rare; most apparently asymptomatic cases probably result from internal (e.g., intravaginal) lesions

Epidemiologic History

- Often commercial sex, illicit drug use, or recent travel to an endemic area
- May appear in discrete outbreaks

PHYSICAL EXAMINATION

- One or more nonindurated genital ulcers with purulent bases
- Males: most common sites are glans, corona, or inner surface of foreskin
- Women: most lesions are at introitus or labia, sometimes intravaginal
- Ulcers usually very tender, but nontender lesions sometimes present
- Surrounding erythema and undermined edges are common
- Multiple ulcers sometimes form "kissing" lesions, with ulceration on apposed surfaces (e.g., under foreskin); said to be pathognomonic for chancroid

- Unilateral or bilateral inguinal lymphadenopathy in 50–60%
- Lymphadenopathy characteristic of pyogenic infection, i.e. overlying erythema, tenderness, often fluctuant, may spontaneously rupture

LABORATORY DIAGNOSIS

- Isolation of *H. ducreyi* from lesion or lymph node aspirate
- Sensitivity of culture 60–80%, depending on specimen management, variations in media, and laboratory's experience
- PCR test available in some research settings, with improved sensitivity compared to culture; commercial PCR or other NAATs may become available
- Gram stain of lymph node aspirate may show small gram-negative bacilli, but is insensitive and nonspecific
- All suspected cases require culture or PCR for HSV and darkfield microscopy and serological testing for syphilis

DIAGNOSTIC CRITERIA

- Identification of *H. ducreyi* by culture or PCR is definitive
- In absence of microbiologic confirmation, diagnosis is based on clinical findings, epidemiologic setting, and exclusion of herpes and syphilis

TREATMENT

Principles

- Resistance to penicillins and tetracyclines is common
- Third-generation cephalosporins are consistently active
- Fluoroquinolones and macrolides generally are active, but sporadic resistance occurs
- Higher clinical failure rates may occur in HIV-infected persons

Recommended Treatments

- Azithromycin 1.0 g PO, single dose
- Ceftriaxone 250 mg IM, single dose

Alternative Treatments

- Ciprofloxacin 500 mg PO *bid* for 3 days
- Erythromycin base 500 mg PO *tid* for 7 days

Partner Management

- Refer, examine, and treat all recent sex partners
- Expedited partner therapy (EPT) has not been studied but is a reasonable option if direct clinical intervention is not feasible

PREVENTION

- Assure referral and treatment of sex partners
- Advise condoms and other elements of sexual safety
- Report cases to local or regional health authorities

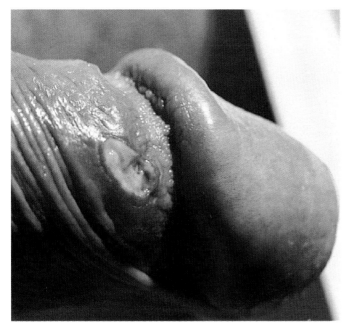

6–1. Chancroidal ulcer of penis.

CASE

Patient Profile Age 26, unmarried salesman

History Painful sore on penis for 5 days; sex 10 days earlier with a female commercial sex worker in a developing country; had sex with regular partner once, before penile lesion noticed

Examination Tender, nonindurated ulcerative penile lesion with purulent base; uncircumcised; no lymphadenopathy

Differential Diagnosis Chancroid, genital herpes, syphilis

Laboratory Stat RPR and darkfield microscopy negative; culture of lesion positive for *H. ducreyi*; culture negative for HSV; urethral tests for *Neisseria gonorrhoeae* and *Chlamydia trachomatis* negative; HIV serology negative

Diagnosis Chancroid

Treatment Azithromycin 1.0 g PO, single dose

Partner Management Current partner had normal examination, with negative vaginal culture for *H. ducreyi*; treated with azithromycin

Comment Lesion pain improved in 2 days, healed by 14 days; patient scheduled for follow-up VDRL and repeat HIV serology 2–3 months later

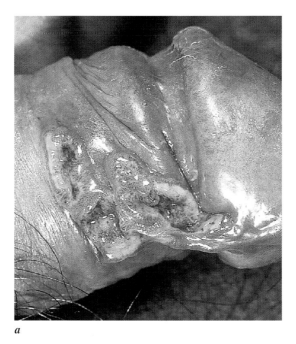

a

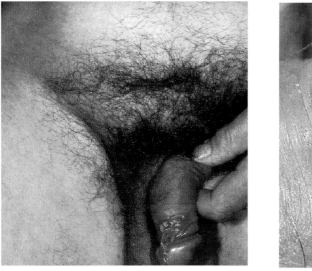

b

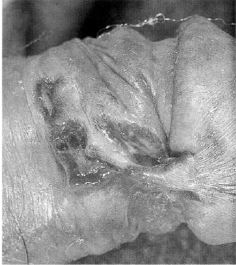

c

6–2. Chancroid. *a.* Large, irregularly shaped penile ulcers under foreskin; the ulceration had perforated the frenulum of the penis, through which a probe could be passed. *b.* Inguinal swelling and erythema extending to lower abdomen. *c.* Healing ulcers 1 week after starting treatment; reduced purulent exudate and partial reepithelialization.

CASE

Patient Profile Age 60, businessman with a large international corporation

History Painful, enlarging penile ulcers for 2 weeks; onset 5 days after sexual exposure in equatorial Africa; painful right inguinal swelling for 3 days; company's occupational medicine clinic prescribed amoxicillin, without improvement after 5 days

Examination Multiple, coalescing, irregularly shaped, purulent tender ulcers under foreskin; 3 × 5-cm indurated, tender, nonfluctuant right inguinal lymph node; inguinal erythema extending to the low abdominal wall

Differential Diagnosis Chancroid; herpes, syphilis, and lymphogranuloma venereum less likely; possible pyogenic infection

Laboratory *H. ducreyi* isolated by culture; darkfield examination, VDRL, culture for HSV (all negative); urethral cultures for *N. gonorrhoeae* and *C. trachomatis* (negative); HIV serology (negative)

Diagnosis Chancroid

Treatment Ceftriaxone 250 mg IM, single dose, followed by amoxicillin with clavulanic acid (Augmentin) 500/125 mg PO *tid* for 10 days

Management of Sex Partners Patient advised to notify his distant partner; he had not resumed intercourse with his wife, who was not informed

Comment Amoxicillin/clavulanic acid was prescribed because the atypically extensive inguinal erythema suggested secondary pyogenic cellulitis. The ulcers healed rapidly and erythema regressed, but the right lymph node became fluctuant and required needle aspiration 10 days after start of treatment. Follow-up VDRL was negative after 1 month, and repeat HIV serology was negative after 1 month and 3 months. At numerous visits to his company's occupational medicine clinic in anticipation of international travel, the patient, who regularly was sexually active with local residents when traveling, was offered appropriate immunizations and malaria prophylaxis and was counseled on avoidance of food-borne illness, but was not asked about plans for sexual activity or advised about condoms or other aspects of safer sex. Pretravel counseling should routinely include inquiry about plans for sex and, when appropriate, STD/HIV prevention advice.

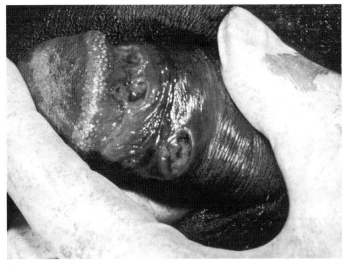

a

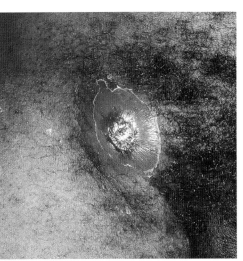

b

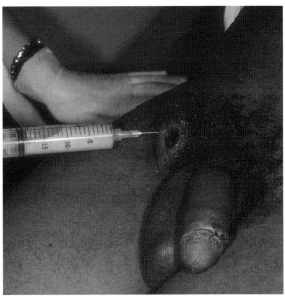

c

6–3. Chancroid in a patient who presented with painful genital ulcers and swelling in the groin that "opened and drained pus" 3 days earlier. *a.* Deeply eroded ulcers under retracted foreskin. (Pearly penile papules also are present.) *b.* Fluctuant lymph node with eschar at site of previous spontaneous rupture and drainage. *c.* Needle aspiration of lymph node.

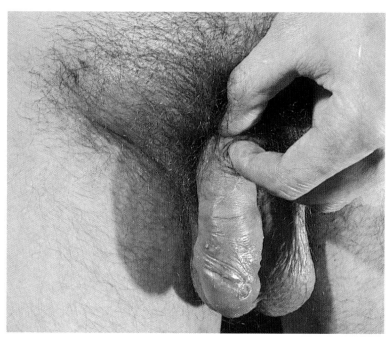

6–4. Chancroid, with penile ulcers and inguinal lymphadenopathy with overlying cutaneous erythema. The small eschars lateral to the lymph node mark the sites of needle aspirations.

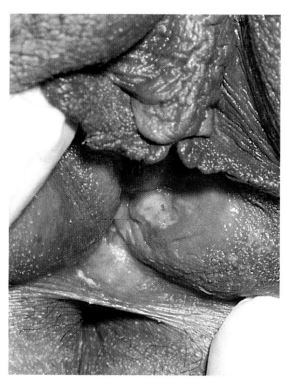

6–5. Chancroidal ulcer of vaginal introitus. (*Reproduced with permission from Holmes KK, et al. Sexually Transmitted Diseases. 3rd ed. New York, NY: McGraw-Hill; 1999.*)

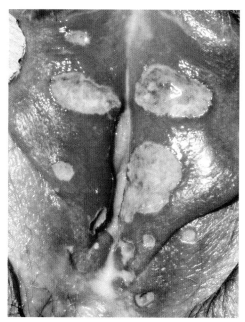

6–6. Multiple introital and labial ulcers in a woman with chancroid. Some lesions illustrate autoinoculation between apposed surfaces, sometimes called "kissing lesions," a classical feature of chancroid. (*Reprinted with permission from Wolff K, Johnson RA. Fitzpatrick's Color Atlas and Synopsis of Clinical Dermatology. 6th ed. New York, NY: McGraw-Hill; 2009.*)

SUGGESTED READING

Janowicz DM, et al. Experimental infection of human volunteers with *Haemophilus ducreyi*: fifteen years of clinical data and experience. *J Infect Dis.* 2009;199:1671-9. *A summary of extensive studies that have contributed immeasurably to understanding of chancroid transmission, clinical manifestations, and pathogenesis.*

Mohammed TT, Olumide YM. Chancroid and human immunodeficiency virus infection: a review. *Int J Dermatol.* 2008;47:1-8. *An erudite review of the epidemiology, clinical manifestations, and interactions of chancroid with HIV/AIDS in Africa.*

Peel TN, et al. Chronic cutaneous ulcers secondary to *Haemophilus ducreyi* infection. *Med J Aust.* 2010;192:248-50. *Report of two cases of nonsexually transmitted chancroid, with review of other reported cases.*

Spinola SM. Chancroid and *Haemophilus ducreyi*. Chapter 39 in KK Holmes, et al., eds. *Sexually Transmitted Diseases.* 4th ed. New York, NY: McGraw-Hill, 2008;689-99. *A comprehensive review by the leading chancroid investigator.*

7

Donovanosis

The indolent genital ulcer disease donovanosis, formerly called granuloma inguinale, is one of the five originally defined venereal diseases (with syphilis, gonorrhea, lymphogranuloma venereum, and chancroid). Donovanosis now is rare worldwide, including some areas where it formerly was endemic, such as Papua New Guinea, Australia, and the Indian subcontinent. A specific donovanosis eradication campaign appears to have been successful in aboriginal populations in Australia. The causative organism, *Calymmatobacterium granulomatis*, is a gram-negative bacillus related to *Klebsiella* species. The organism was only recently grown in sustained culture, but diagnosis remains dependent largely on clinical and histologic criteria. A polymerase chain reaction (PCR) test has been developed and this or other nucleic acid amplification tests (NAATs) may become available in the future. Sexual transmission is surmised by genital localization and occasional disease in infected persons' sex partners, but most partners are free of clinical disease. A colonic reservoir and transmission by fecal contamination of abraded skin have been hypothesized. The disease may progress slowly for several years, with locally destructive outcomes that mimic those of cutaneous cancer. Several antibiotics are believed to be effective, although no well-controlled trials are available.

EPIDEMIOLOGY

Incidence and Prevalence

- Rare in the United States and industrialized countries and increasingly rare in developing countries; largely limited to isolated populations with irregular health care
- No reported cases in the United States since 2000
- Most cases in industrialized countries are imported from endemic areas

Transmission

- Probably by sexual contact, but most sex partners apparently are uninfected
- Some cases may be transmitted by nonsexual routes, perhaps by fecal contact with abraded skin
- Occasional perinatal transmission to newborns

Age

- No known predilection

Sex

- In endemic areas, cases in men typically outnumber those in women, perhaps related to exposure patterns (e.g., commercial sex)

Sexual Orientation

- No known predisposition
- Few cases reported in homosexual men or women, perhaps due in part to reduced recognition of homosexuality in endemic areas

HISTORY

Incubation Period

- Usually 2–3 weeks, perhaps up to 1 year

Symptoms

- Slowly progressive mucocutaneous ulceration that may become extensive
- Usually painless
- Occasional multiple lesions
- Occasional inguinal swelling
- Rare local symptoms of disseminated osteomyelitis
- Generally no fever or other systemic symptoms

Epidemiologic History

- Residency or sexual exposure in an endemic area

PHYSICAL EXAMINATION

- Four clinical variants:
  - Ulcerogranulomatous: hypertrophic red granulation tissue with easily induced bleeding
  - Hypertrophic: exuberant exophytic, wart-like ("verruciform") lesions
  - Necrotic: deep ulceration, extensive tissue destruction
  - Sclerotic: prominent fibrosis, sometimes with urethral stricture
- Little or no purulent exudate; pus may indicate secondary infection
- Usually involves penis or vulva; sometimes perianal; occasional nongenital sites
- Inguinal mass ("pseudobubo") may result from subcutaneous extension of inflammatory tissue; usually no true lymphadenopathy
- Extensive ulceration can persist and progress several years, mimicking cancer; penile autoamputation has been observed

- Rare systemic dissemination, with hepatic or osteolytic lesions
- Cervical lymphadenitis has occurred in young children

LABORATORY DIAGNOSIS

- Histologic identification of organism in vacuoles within macrophages ("Donovan bodies") using modified Giemsa stain of biopsied tissue or crush preparation
- PCR assay has been described, not yet commercially available

DIAGNOSTIC CRITERIA

- Based primarily on clinical presentation and exclusion of alternate diagnosis
- Biopsy or crush preparation showing characteristic histopathology
- Exposure history in endemic area

TREATMENT

Principles

- Antimicrobial susceptibility uncertain; surmised primarily by clinical response to empirical therapy
- Treat for 3 weeks to 3 months, until healed
- Longer treatment may be required in HIV-infected patients

Recommended Regimen

- Doxycycline 100 mg PO *bid* for 3 weeks to 3 months

Alternative Regimens

- Azithromycin 1.0 g PO once weekly
- Ciprofloxacin 750 mg PO *bid*
- Erythromycin base 500 mg PO *qid*
- Trimethoprim/sulfamethoxazole 800 mg/160 mg PO *bid*

PREVENTION AND CONTROL

- Identify and offer treatment to sex partners
- Value of treatment for partners without clinically evident infection is unknown

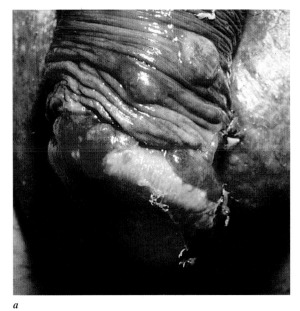
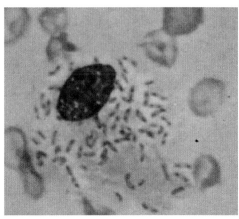

a   *b*

7–1. Donovanosis, ulcerogranulomatous variety. *a.* Penile lesions. *b.* Giemsa stain of crush preparation of tissue from penile lesion, showing a macrophage with vacuoles containing bipolar-staining bacilli (Donovan bodies). (*Courtesy of Gavin Hart, M.D.*)

CASE

Patient Profile Age 47, merchant seaman

History Painless penile sores for 3 weeks; during 2 months prior to onset had unprotected commercial sex in South Asian seaport cities

Examination Multiple, slightly tender, hypertrophic ulcerative penile lesions; no lymphadenopathy

Differential Diagnosis Donovanosis, primary syphilis, cancer

Laboratory Giemsa stain of crush preparation of biopsy specimen showed large mononuclear cells with Donovan bodies; darkfield examination, lesion cultures for HSV and *Haemophilus ducreyi*, VDRL, HIV serology (all negative)

Diagnosis Donovanosis

Treatment Doxycycline 100 mg PO *bid* for 3 weeks

Follow-up Lesions had regressed and were partly reepithelialized after 10 days, after which patient was lost to follow-up

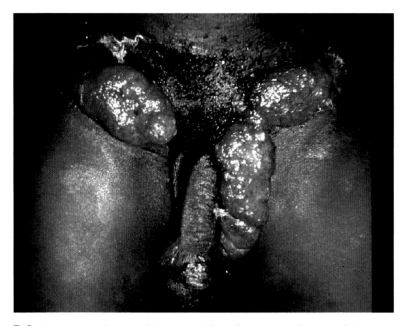

7–2. Donovanosis, hypertrophic variety, with exuberant granulomatous lesions. *(Reproduced with permission from Holmes KK, et al. Sexually Transmitted Diseases. 3rd ed. New York, NY: McGraw-Hill; 1999.)*

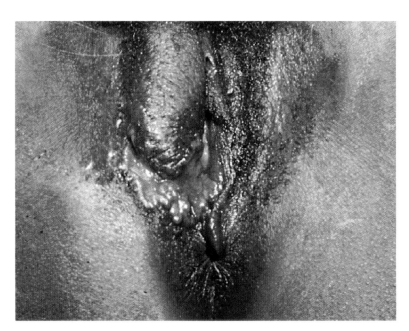

7–3. Donovanosis with features of both ulcerogranulomatous and necrotic varieties, with extensive genital ulceration and vulvar lymphedema. *(Reproduced with permission from Holmes KK, et al. Sexually Transmitted Diseases. 3rd ed. New York,NY: McGraw-Hill; 1999.)*

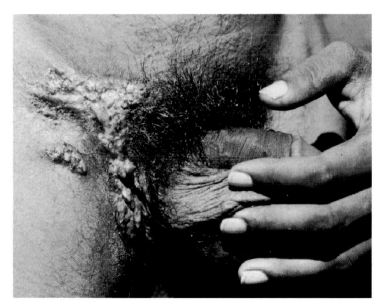

7–4. Donovanosis, sclerotic variety, with hypertrophic verruciform lesions. (*Reproduced with permission from Holmes KK, et al. Sexually Transmitted Diseases. 3rd ed. New York, NY: McGraw-Hill; 1999.*)

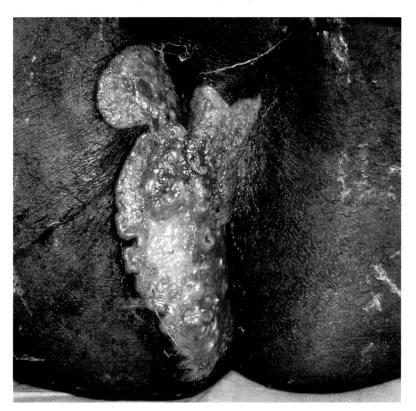

7-5. Donovanosis. Extensive hypertrophic ulceration and scarring of the intragluteal cleft, perineum, and scrotum. (*Reprinted with permission from Wolff K, Johnson RA. Fitzpatrick's Color Atlas and Synopsis of Clinical Dermatology. 6th ed. New York, NY: McGraw-Hill; 2009.*)

SUGGESTED READING

O'Farrell N. Donovanosis. Chapter 40 in KK Holmes, et al., eds. *Sexually Transmitted Diseases.* 4th ed. New York, NY: McGraw-Hill; 2008:701-8. *A comprehensive review by a leading authority on donovanosis.*

Viral Sexually Transmitted Diseases

8

Genital Herpes

Genital herpes is the most common cause of genital ulceration in most countries, with an estimated incidence in the United States up to one million cases per year and a prevalence of 50 to 60 million persons. Most cases of recurrent genital herpes are caused by herpes simplex virus type 2 (HSV-2), but up to half of all initial genital infections are due to HSV type 1 (HSV-1), the usual cause of orolabial herpes. Infection with either HSV type is lifelong, with virus persisting in neural tissue, especially the cranial or dorsal spinal nerve root ganglia, and at infected mucocutaneous sites. The presence of specific antibody denotes current infection and the potential for clinical recurrences, subclinical viral shedding, and transmission to sex partners. HSV infections have long been viewed as mostly latent with relatively infrequent reactivation. However, recent research shows unapparent viral replication to be much more frequent than previously understood, and herpes is more accurately characterized as a continuously active infection than a recurrent one.

Both symptomatic and asymptomatic recurrences are substantially more frequent for genital HSV-2 than for genital or oral HSV-1. Almost all genital HSV-2 infections are acquired by genital or anal intercourse, whereas most genital HSV-1 infections are acquired by orogenital exposure. Because of the reduced recurrence frequency, genital to genital HSV-1 transmission probably is uncommon. Therefore, HSV-2 seroprevalence in a population accurately denotes genital infection, whereas HSV-1 antibody reflects orolabial infection plus a substantial (albeit unquantified) proportion with genital herpes. Owing to varied clinical manifestations, complexity of diagnosis, multiple treatment options, multifaceted prevention strategies, and the need for sophisticated counseling, the clinical management of genital herpes is more complex than that of any STD except HIV/AIDS.

Most genital HSV infections are subclinical, but many apparently asymptomatic persons have mild or nonspecific symptoms whose significance is not understood until infection is suspected by transmission to a partner or through serological testing. No cure exists, but therapy with acyclovir and related drugs accelerates healing of lesions and reduces the frequencies of recurrent outbreaks, asymptomatic reactivation, and sexual transmission of HSV-2. The most common serious complication is perinatal transmission resulting in neonatal herpes, which often is fatal or causes permanent neurodevelopmental sequelae. Other biomedical complications in adults include meningitis (primarily HSV-2), encephalitis (mostly due to HSV-1), aggressive and persistent mucocutaneous ulceration in persons with AIDS or other immune deficiencies, erythema multiforme, Stevens Johnson syndrome, and rare cases of systemic dissemination with hepatic necrosis which often is fatal. Herpetic whitlow and keratoconjunctivitis can result from auto-inoculation during initial and less commonly during recurrent herpes. The psychological impact of genital herpes also can be substantial, primarily resulting from fear of transmission to sex partners.

As for all inflammatory STDs, HSV-2 infection (but apparently not HSV-1, whether oral or genital) is associated with enhanced sexual acquisition of HIV, even when asymptomatic. Owing to the high prevalence of HSV-2 in almost all populations at risk for HIV, genital herpes has greater population-level impact on HIV transmission than all other STDs, accounting for up to half of all HIV infections worldwide. Unfortunately, however, treatment of HSV-2 infected persons with acyclovir does not reduce the risk of HIV infection. At least part of the explanation appears to be frequent viral replication and a subclinical inflammatory response that persist at mucosal and cutaneous sites of recurrent outbreaks regardless of antiviral therapy, which includes activated lymphocytes and dendritic cells that are especially susceptible to HIV.

The priority that should be accorded prevention efforts against genital and neonatal herpes is controversial, as is serological screening for HSV-2 in persons at risk. However, there is no debate about the diagnostic utility of HSV type-specific serological tests or viral detection by culture or polymerase chain reaction (PCR) in patients with genital herpes or genital ulcer disease. Virus type should be determined in all patients with genital herpes, because of the differences between genital HSV-1 and HSV-2 infection in clinical course, the potential for sexual transmission, and susceptibility to HIV.

EPIDEMIOLOGY

Incidence and Prevalence

- National seroprevalence of HSV-2 antibody in 14- to 49-year-old U.S. residents was 16% in 2005–2008, stable since 2001–2004 (17%)
- About 45 million persons in the United States are infected with HSV-2; the total with genital herpes, including HSV-1, probably exceeds 60 million
- Initial visits to physicians for genital herpes rose from ~100,000 per year in 1970s to ~300,000 annually in 2006–2009
- In western Europe, HSV-2 seroprevalence is generally lower than in United States; 10–15% in most countries
- HSV-2 seroprevalence is ≥50% in many developing countries
- HSV-1 seroprevalence (mostly reflecting orolabial infection) is 50–90% in adults in most countries

Transmission

- Requires direct contact with infected tissues or secretions
- Most genital infections are acquired from partners with subclinical infection
- Prior infection apparently confers resistance, if not complete immunity, to reinfection with the same HSV type at any anatomic location

- ○ Superinfections with same virus type uncommon
- ○ Mutually infected sexually active couples do not reinfect one another
- Autoinoculation can result in herpetic whitlow or keratoconjunctivitis
  - ○ Mostly during primary infections
  - ○ Rare in persons with longstanding, recurrent herpes
- No documented transmission by fomites, shared clothing or towels, or environmental exposure (e.g., toilets), notwithstanding occasional assertions by patients or face-saving explanations by naïve clinicians
- Perinatal transmission to newborns, especially following new infection in late pregnancy

Age

- In the United States in 2005–2008, HSV-2 seroprevalence was 1% at age 14–19, 10.5% at age 20–29, 20% at age 30–39, 26% at age 40–49
- All ages are susceptible, but in the United States genital HSV-2 is acquired most frequently by persons age 25–35 years

Sex

- Women are more susceptible to genital HSV than men, owing to larger surface area exposed and increased mucosal exposure
- National seroprevalence of HSV-2 in the United States in 2005–2008 was 21% in women, 12% in men

Sexual Orientation

- MSM generally higher HSV-2 seroprevalence than age-comparable heterosexual men (e.g. 25–30%)

Other Risk Factors

- Race/ethnicity: HSV-2 seroprevalence in the United States during 2005–2008:
  - ○ African Americans, 39%
  - ○ Whites, 12%
  - ○ Mexican Americans, 10%
- Independent of race, HSV-2 and HSV-1 prevalences are highest in lower socioeconomic populations

CLINICAL CLASSIFICATION

Primary Genital Herpes

- Definition: Patient's first infection with either HSV type
- Seronegative at onset for both HSV-1 and HSV-2
- Symptomatic cases commonly are severe, often prolonged (3–4 weeks) if untreated
- Frequent mucosal involvement (e.g., cervicitis, urethritis), regional lymphadenopathy, regional neuropathy, fever, headache, malaise
- Up to 50% of cases due to HSV-1, acquired primarily by orogenital exposure

- Evolution from initial papule to crust and healing typically requires 10–15 days for initial herpes, 7–10 days for reactivations
- Recurrent lesions typically occur in clusters, but single lesions are common
- Recurrent lesion locations:
  - Usually genitals (penis, introitus, labia, vulva) or perigenital areas (e.g., anus, perineum)
  - Can occur in any sacral nerve distribution, e.g. buttocks, upper things, lower abdomen, hip, etc. ("boxer shorts" area)
- Lesions generally not associated with hairs (vs. folliculitis)
- Ulcers usually tender, nonindurated
- Lesions may be small, "nonspecific" in appearance, mimicking excoriation and other noninfectious conditions
- Lymphadenopathy, when present, usually is bilateral, firm, moderately tender, without fluctuance or cutaneous erythema
- Erosive cervicitis in ≥50% of women with primary herpes; overt cervicitis uncommon in reactivation
- Urethritis in 30–40% of men with primary herpes, often meatal erythema and/or localized tenderness along penile shaft at sites of intraurethral lesions (see Chap. 16)
- Occasional sacral nerve neurological deficits in primary infection (e.g., urinary retention, lax anal sphincter)
- Deeply erosive genital, perianal, or perioral lesions are common in AIDS patients
- Signs of meningitis, e.g., nuchal rigidity, photophobia
- Erythema multiforme is an occasional systemic response to recurrent genital herpes

LABORATORY DIAGNOSIS

Diagnostic Principles

- Diagnosis in all suspected cases should be virologically confirmed and HSV type determined
- Identification of HSV in lesion by PCR or culture is definitive; negative result usually does not exclude herpes
- Type-specific HSV antibody testing often is diagnostically useful in patients with atypical or culture-negative lesions or who present without current lesions; seroconversion is diagnostically definitive
- Rule out syphilis, chancroid, and other causes of genital ulcer by epidemiologic assessment and appropriate laboratory tests
- Differential of genital ulcer disease includes traumatic lesions (e.g., excoriation in presence of pruritic syndromes), folliculitis, fissures caused by vulvovaginal candidiasis, aphthous ulcers, Behçet disease, ulceration due to erythema multiforme (Stevens Johnson syndrome), and other causes

Virologic Tests
Culture

- Isolation in cell culture is available in most clinical laboratories in industrialized countries
- Yield highest in initial episodes or from recurrent lesions ≤2 days old

Nucleic Acid Amplification Tests

- Test of choice when available; more sensitive than culture
- PCR and other NAATs are increasingly available in the United States and other industrialized countries

Other Tests

- Direct fluorescence microscopy for HSV less sensitive and does not differentiate HSV-1 from HSV-2; little clinical utility
- Cytologic identification of multinucleated giant cells (Tzanck test) is pathognomonic for herpes but is insensitive and does not differentiate HSV-1, HSV-1, or varicella zoster virus

Serology

- Type-specific tests, based on antibody specific to HSV glycoprotein G1 (for HSV-1) or glycoprotein G2 (for HSV-2)
  ◦ HerpeSelect IgG HSV-1 and HSV-2 ELISA or immunoblot (Focus Diagnostics)
  ◦ Captia IgG HSV-1 and HSV-2 ELISA (Trinity Biotech)
  ◦ BiokitUSA HSV-2 rapid point-of care test (Biokit USA)
  ◦ Kalon HSV-1 and HSV-2 ELISA (available in the United Kingdom and other countries)
  ◦ Several other assays now available in various countries and more are anticipated
- IgG HSV-2 ELISA (HerpeSelect) performance characteristics
  ◦ Optical density ratio >1.1 formally defines positive result
  ◦ Values 1.1–3.5 may be false positive and require repeat or confirmatory testing
  ◦ Values ≥3.5 are definitely positive
- Intermediate results have not been systematically studied for tests other than HerpeSelect; repeat or confirm positive results that do not accord with clinical manifestations or risk assessment
- HSV Western blot is serological gold standard; final arbiter of uncertain test results requiring confirmation
- An ELISA inhibition assay (Focus Diagnostics) may be useful for confirmation, but may not be commercially available
- Non-type-specific antibody tests
  ◦ May be used for inexpensive initial testing; negative result excludes HSV-1 and HSV-2; positive result requires follow-up type-specific test
  ◦ Numerous tests marketed worldwide falsely claim to be type-specific; avoid tests that do not explicitly detect antibody to HSV glycoproteins G1 and G2
- HSV-2 seroconversion
  ◦ IgG HSV-2 antibody (e.g., HerpeSelect): ~50% of newly infected patients seropositive at 3–4 weeks, 70–80% at 6–8 weeks, ≥90% at 3 months
  ◦ Seroconversion is slower for Western blot: ~50% at 6–8 weeks, 80% at 3 months, ≥90% at 1 year
  ◦ Seroconversion time not well studied for most other assays

- ~5% of persons with HSV-2 infections and ~15% with HSV-1 do not develop detectable type-specific antibody and have persistently false-negative results
- Antiviral therapy of initial HSV infection may delay or prevent seroconversion
- IgM antibody testing
  - Measurable IgM antibody to HSV often does not precede IgG and IgM can persist in recurrent herpes; therefore, positive IgM test does not reliably indicate infection
  - False-positive results are common
  - All IgM tests are non-type-specific
  - Therefore, IgM testing is rarely useful in clinical diagnosis of either initial or recurrent infection; routine IgM testing is not recommended

TREATMENT

Antiviral Therapy Principles

- Oral acyclovir, valacyclovir, or famciclovir are mainstays of treatment
- Valacyclovir and famciclovir are "pro-drugs", i.e., converted to acyclovir and penciclovir during absorption
- Side effects and allergy are rare
- Treatment substantially speeds clinical resolution of initial herpes; lesser benefit for recurrent outbreaks
- Topical acyclovir or penciclovir has little clinical effect, rarely indicated
- HSV drug resistance is rare
  - Primarily occurs in immunodeficient patients after prolonged or repeated drug exposure
  - Alternative therapies include foscarnet, cidofovir, and topical trifluridine

Recommended Regimens

Initial (Primary and Nonprimary) Genital Herpes

All cases should be treated, even if apparently mild, to shorten duration of symptoms and prevent accelerated course. Even with prompt clinical response, relapse can occur if treatment is stopped early.

- Valacyclovir 1.0 g PO *bid* for 7–10 days
- Acyclovir 400 mg PO *tid* for 7–10 days
- Famciclovir 250 mg PO *tid* for 7–10 days
- Severe cases requiring parenteral therapy: acyclovir 5–10 mg/kg body weight IV every 8 hours for 5–7 days or until improved, then oral valacyclovir, acyclovir, or famciclovir to complete 10–14 days total

Recurrent Genital Herpes

Suppressive therapy is generally preferable to episodic treatment of individual recurrences. Suppression reduces symptomatic HSV-2 recurrences by 70–80% and in a randomized controlled trial valacyclovir reduced the frequency of sexual transmission by 48%; owing to aspects of study design, actual prevention efficacy may be higher. Acyclovir has not been studied for prevention of transmission but may have efficacy similar to valacyclovir. Famciclovir is somewhat less effective than valacyclovir in suppressing symptomatic recurrences and subclinical shedding. The option of suppressive therapy should be routinely discussed and offered to all patients with genital HSV-2 to help prevent sexual transmission and reduce the frequency of symptomatic reactivation; it is especially indicated for those with ≥6 outbreaks per year, clinically severe outbreaks, or significant psychological impact of recurrent herpes. The efficacy of suppressive therapy has not been studied in genital HSV-1 infection and is less frequently indicated in such patients, owing to typically low frequencies of reactivation. Suppressive treatment may be interrupted periodically (e.g., at 1–2 year intervals) to reassess frequency and severity of outbreaks. Some experts recommend that suppressive therapy be deferred for several months after initial diagnosis of genital herpes in order to assess the frequency and severity of recurrent outbreaks unaffected by antiviral treatment and reduce the possibility of delayed seroconversion. However, delayed treatment may be impractical in patients with new or susceptible sex partners, or for patients with severe psychological impact of newly acquired infection. Episodic therapy is preferred by some patients and speeds healing of recurrent outbreaks by 1–2 days if started within 1 day of onset, and patients with prodrome may abort mucocutaneous outbreaks by prompt treatment. Effective episodic therapy requires prior prescription so that patients have drug available for immediate self-treatment.

Suppressive Treatment

- Valacyclovir 500 mg PO once daily; or 1.0 g PO once daily if ≥10 symptomatic outbreaks per year
  - It is plausible, but unproved, that 1.0 g daily may be more effective than 500 mg daily in preventing transmission, regardless of recurrence frequency
- Acyclovir 400 mg PO *bid*
- Famciclovir 250 mg PO *bid*

Episodic Treatment

- Valacyclovir 500 mg PO *bid* for 3 days
- Valacyclovir 1.0 g PO once daily for 5 days
- Acyclovir 800 mg PO *tid* for 2 days
- Acyclovir 800 mg PO *bid* for 5 days
- Acyclovir 400 mg PO *tid* for 5 days
- Famciclovir 1.0 g PO, 2 doses 12 hours apart
- Famciclovir 500 mg PO once, then 250 mg PO *bid* for 2 days
- Famciclovir 125 mg PO *bid* for 5 days

Supportive Therapy

- Keep lesions clean and dry by washing 2–3 times daily and wearing loosely fitting cotton underwear
- Topical anesthetic ointment may help control pain, especially in initial genital herpes

Management of Sex Partners

- Evaluate partners not known to have genital herpes
  - Type-specific serological test to diagnose subclinical infection and determine susceptibility to infection
  - Examine partners promptly (within 1–2 days) if symptoms of herpes appear

Counseling

Advise patient and partner(s) about:

- Available prevention strategies (see Prevention)
- Likelihood of recurrences, frequency of subclinical shedding, and potential for transmission, including differences between HSV-1 and HSV-2
- Elevated risk and frequency of recurrent outbreaks, subclinical viral shedding, and transmission in first 6 months after initial infection
- Routine disclosure of genital HSV-2 to prospective new sex partners
- Methods to minimize impact of genital herpes on current and new sexual relationships
- Importance of not allowing herpes to substantially affect current or future committed sexual relationships
  - Likelihood of mild or subclinical infection in partner if transmission occurs despite attempts to prevent it
  - Treatment available in event of significant symptoms
  - Main fear of genital herpes is transmission to new partners, generally not a concern in committed relationships
- Elevated risk of HIV infection if sexually exposed
- Risks and prevention of neonatal herpes
- During initial infection, avoidance of autoinoculation and resultant herpetic keratitis or whitlow
  - Minimize manual contact with lesions
  - Frequent hand washing or alcohol gel
  - Autoinoculation is rare in recurrent or long-established HSV infection
- Rarity of HSV transmission in households, by fomites, or from contaminated surfaces; household members (other than sex partners) are not at risk

PREVENTION

Genital Herpes

- Transmission risk is low, perhaps zero, to partners infected with the same HSV type; partners can be serologically tested to assess susceptibility
- Disclosure of genital herpes to uninfected partners is associated with reduced transmission risk

- Condoms for vaginal or anal sex
  - Reduces HSV-2 transmission risk by ≥90% for individual episodes of vaginal intercourse
  - Long-term efficacy (use effectiveness) to prevent HSV-2 transmission probably 50–70%
- Suppressive therapy
  - Valacyclovir reduces HSV-2 transmission risk by ≥50%
  - Acyclovir probably has similar efficacy
  - Famciclovir is less effective in suppressing viral shedding and may be less effective in preventing transmission
- Avoid sex during symptomatic reactivations, from prodrome until healed
- Transmission probably is uncommon when all three strategies (condoms, suppressive therapy, avoiding sex during outbreaks) are used

Neonatal Herpes

- Highest risk is from maternal initial genital infection in third trimester; accounts for ~50% of neonatal herpes
- Serological testing of pregnant women and, if seronegative, their sex partners may help prevent neonatal herpes by identifying discordant couples and counseling them to avoid intercourse or orogenital exposure (depending on HSV type) in third trimester
- Cesarean section for women with clinically apparent herpes lesions at term
- HSV PCR with rapid results (<4 hours) is useful during labor; consider cesarean delivery for suspected initial infection, i.e., patient seronegative to the HSV type identified by PCR
- In recurrent genital herpes, prophylactic acyclovir during last month of pregnancy prevents otherwise unnecessary cesarean deliveries by reducing frequency of symptomatic reactivation; efficacy for preventing perinatal transmission is unknown

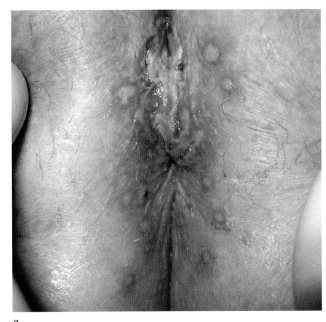

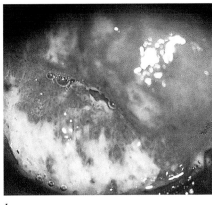

8–1. Primary genital herpes. *a.* Multiple, bilateral ulcers of vulva, anus, perineum, and buttocks. *b.* Ulcerative cervicitis. (*Part b courtesy of Claire E. Stevens.*)

a

b

CASE

Patient Profile Age 22, single secretary

History Genital and perianal pain, vaginal discharge, fever, and headache for 7 days; boyfriend has recurrent genital herpes, but they carefully avoided sex during symptomatic episodes

Examination Multiple bilateral tender ulcers of labia and medial aspects of buttocks; ulcers and purulent exudate of cervix; tender inguinal lymphadenopathy bilaterally; temperature 38.1°C orally

Differential Diagnosis Genital herpes, contact dermatitis; syphilis and chancroid unlikely

Laboratory HSV-2 isolated from lesions and cervix; syphilis serology, HIV serology, screening NAATs for *Chlamydia trachomatis* and *Neisseria gonorrhoeae* (all negative)

Diagnosis Primary genital herpes

Treatment Valacyclovir 1.0 g PO *bid* for 10 days

Comment Primary infection (i.e., likely seronegative for HSV-1) is suggested by extensive lesions, inguinal lymphadenopathy, cervicitis, and systemic manifestations. The patient reported substantial pain relief after 3 days and her lesions were completely healed after 2 weeks. She was counseled about likelihood of both symptomatic recurrences and subclinical shedding, with risk of transmission to future sex partners (but not to her current boyfriend). Her partner was examined and counseled; he was unaware about subclinical viral shedding and transmission risk between symptomatic reactivations.

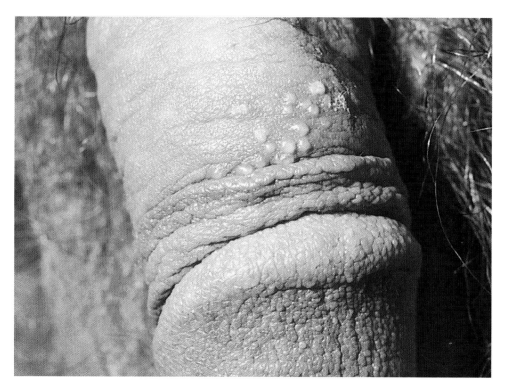

8–2. Cluster of vesicular lesions typical of recurrent genital herpes of 2–3 days duration.

CASE

Patient Profile Age 38, radiology technician

History Penile "blisters" for 2 days, preceded by itching 1 day; two previous similar episodes since initial genital herpes, diagnosed clinically 8 months previously without laboratory confirmation

Examination Cluster of vesicular lesions of penis; no lymphadenopathy

Diagnosis Recurrent genital herpes

Laboratory HSV-2 isolated from lesions

Treatment Valacyclovir 500 mg PO daily as suppressive therapy

Comment Although clinical diagnosis per se did not require laboratory confirmation, viral culture or PCR was indicated to determine virus type. Pain and pruritus resolved over 3 days; the lesions became pustular, then crusted, and healed over 10 days. The patient was counseled about options of episodic or suppressive antiviral therapy, chose the latter, and was symptom-free for the next 6 months.

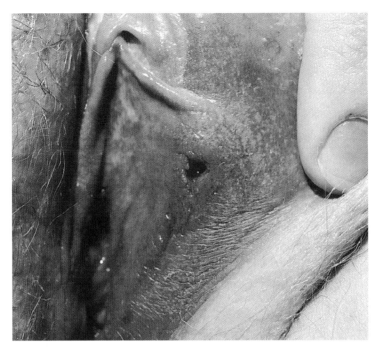

8–3. Genital herpes: subclinical ulcerative lesion of labia minor, with mild surrounding edema.

CASE

Patient Profile Age 28, flight attendant

History Asymptomatic; sought health care after a partner informed her that he had gonorrhea

Examination Nontender ulcer of labia minor, with slight surrounding edema and faint erythema; otherwise normal

Differential Diagnosis Herpes, syphilis, chancroid, traumatic lesion

Laboratory HSV-2 identified in lesion by PCR; darkfield microscopy negative for *Treponema pallidum*; type-specific serology positive for antibody to HSV-2; syphilis and HIV serologies negative; cervical NAAT positive for *N. gonorrhoeae* and *C. trachomatis*

Diagnosis Subclinical recurrent genital herpes; uncomplicated gonorrrhea and chlamydial infection

Treatment Patient elected suppressive therapy with valacyclovir 500 mg PO daily, primarily to prevent transmission to sex partners; ceftriaxone 250 mg IM (single dose), azithromycin 1.0 g PO (single dose)

Comment This case illustrates unrecognized but not truly asymptomatic recurrent genital herpes, which was diagnosed serendipitously when she presented for care because of exposure to gonorrhea. Although the patient initially denied symptoms suggestive of herpes, after palpating the lesion she recalled previous intermittent awareness of a painless swelling in the same spot. Presence of HSV-2 antibody was consistent with chronic infection.

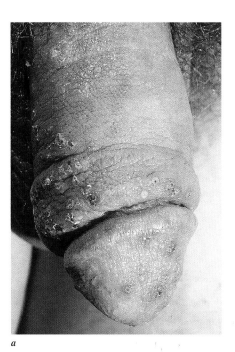

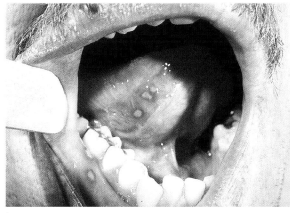

8–4. Primary genital and oral herpes of 1 week duration: *a.* Pustular and crusted lesions of penis, with penile edema. *b.* Oral ulcers. HSV-2 was isolated from both genital and oral lesions. The patient also complained of severe sore throat and fever. When oral HSV-2 infection is seen, it usually accompanies primary genital herpes. Oral HSV-2 rarely causes symptomatic recurrences and asymptomatic oral viral shedding is infrequent.

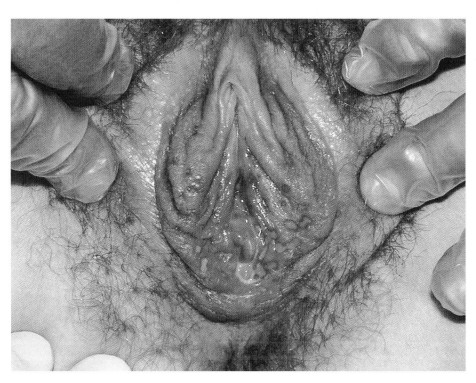

8–5. Primary genital herpes with multiple ulcers of introitus and labia minor. Initial herpes lesions tend to be most prominent at sites of maximum friction during sex. (*Courtesy of Michael L. Remington.*)

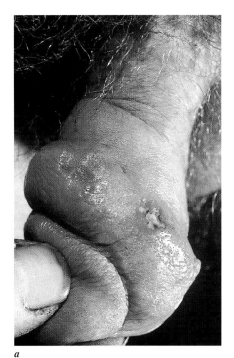

a

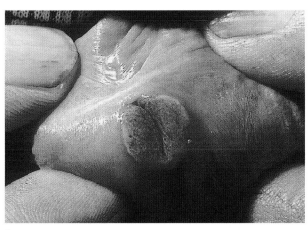

b

8–6. Primary genital herpes: *a.* Ulcerative lesions with penile edema; penile venereal edema can accompany urethritis as well as herpes (also see Figs. 8–4a, 4–8, and 15–4). *b.* Urethritis with meatal ulceration in the same patient; urethritis occurs in about one-third of men with primary genital herpes, often with meatal erythema and severe dysuria, sometimes the only manifestation of herpes (see Chap. 15).

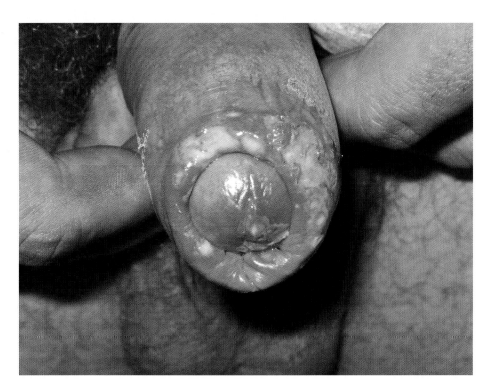

8–7. Primary genital herpes with multiple ulcers of foreskin and glans penis. *(Courtesy of Michael L. Remington.)*

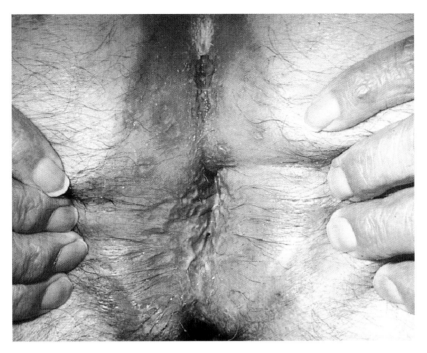

8–8. Primary anal herpes in a gay man. The patient also had fever and tenesmus, and anoscopy showed ulcerative proctitis. HSV-2 was isolated.

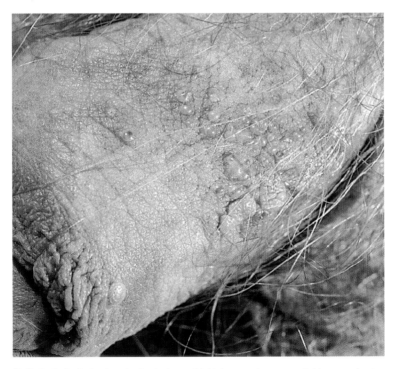

8–9. Early (1–2 days) vesicular lesions of initial, nonprimary genital herpes due to HSV-2 in a patient who was seropositive for HSV-1. Clear fluid-filled vesicles with erythema have been described as "a dew drop on a rose petal," pathognomonic for herpes, including chickenpox and shingles. The patient also has penile warts.

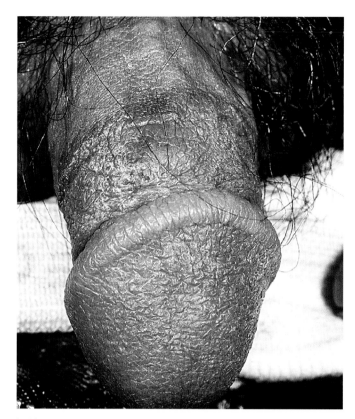

8–10. "Nonspecific" superficial ulcerative lesion due to subclinical recurrent herpes. The patient was asymptomatic until found to be HSV-2-seropositive and counseled to be alert for previously unrecognized lesions.

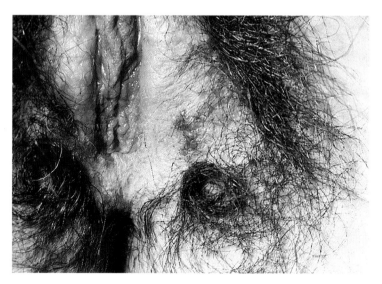

8–11. "Nonspecific" labial ulcer resembling an excoriation in recurrent genital herpes. Many recurrent herpes lesions lack the vesiculopustular characteristics of classic herpes, perhaps especially when observed ≥2 days after onset or if lesion is scratched or manipulated.

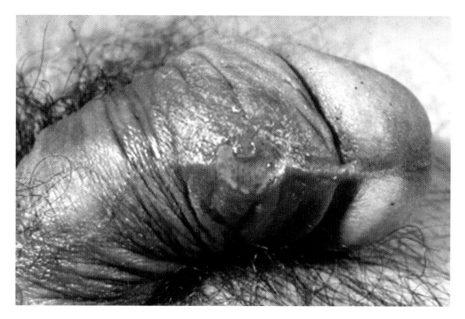

8–12. Initial genital herpes with a single large penile ulcer mimicking chancroid.

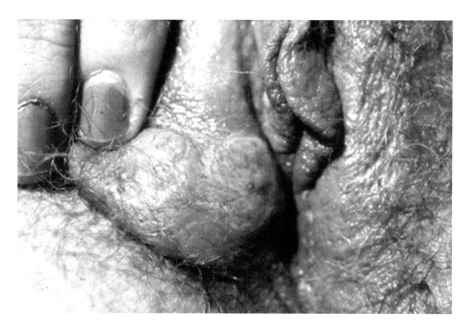

8–13. Large labial ulcers in a woman with initial genital herpes, mimicking chancroid. The labium was edematous and had become bifurcated, so that the two ulcers were in apposition to one another. Autoinoculation across apposed surfaces ("kissing lesions") is considered a classic sign of chancroid but can also occur in initial genital herpes.

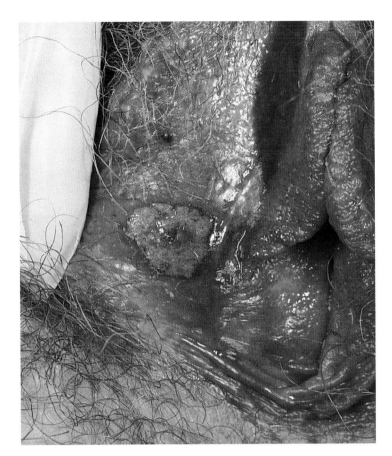

8–14. Initial, nonprimary genital herpes, with a single labial ulcer. The violaceous nodule anterior to the ulcer is a hemangioma.

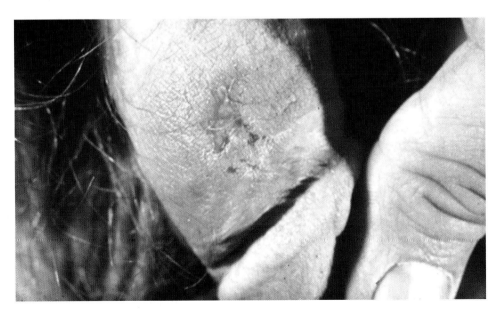

8–15. Irregular, nonspecific-appearing penile ulcer in a man with recurrent genital herpes.

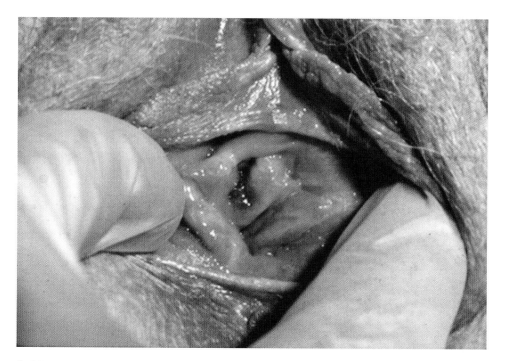

8–16. Initial genital herpes in a woman whose only symptom was dysuria, mimicking a urinary tract infection. Edema surrounds the meatus and the urethra mucosa is ulcerated.

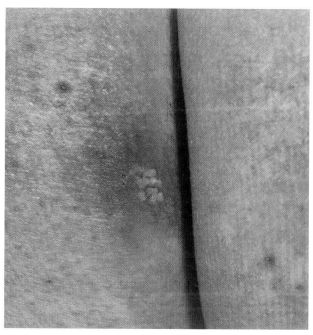

8–17. Recurrent herpes, with a cluster of vesiculopustular lesions in the gluteal cleft.

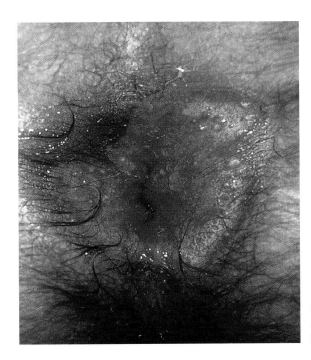

8–18. Chronic erosive perianal herpes of several weeks duration in a man with AIDS (also see Fig. 11–4).

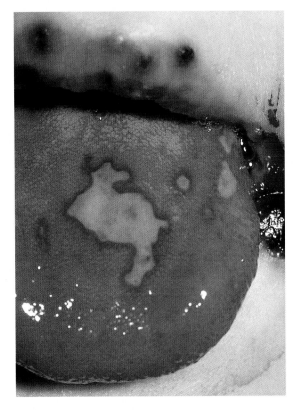

8–19. Gingivostomatitis and vesicular lesions of upper lip in an infant with neonatal herpes. (*Reprinted with permission from Wolff K, Johnson RA. Fitzpatrick's Color Atlas and Synopsis of Clinical Dermatology. 6th ed. New York, NY: McGraw-Hill; 2009.*)

SUGGESTED READING

Brankin AE, et al. Aetiology of genital ulcer disease in female partners of male participants in a circumcision trial in Uganda. *Int J STD AIDS* 2009;20:650-1. *Documentation of HSV as the dominant cause of genital ulcer disease in southern Africa.*

Centers for Disease Control and Prevention. Seroprevalence of herpes simplex virus type 2 among persons aged 14-49 years–United States, 2005-2008. *MMWR.* 2010;59:456-9. http://www.cdc.gov/mmwr/preview/mmwrhtml/mm5915a3.htm. Accessed January 4, 2011. *A periodic CDC report on HSV prevalence, with links to similar reports on HSV-1 seroprevalence.*

Corey L, et al. Once daily valacyclovir to reduce the risk of transmission of genital herpes. *N Engl J Med.* 2004;350:11-20. *The results of a double-blind, placebo-controlled randomized controlled trial demonstrating protection against HSV-2 transmission by valacyclovir.*

Corey L, Wald A. Genital herpes. Chapter 24 in KK Holmes, et al, eds. *Sexually Transmitted Diseases.* 4th ed. New York, NY: McGraw-Hill; 2008:399-437. *A comprehensive, extensively referenced review by two of the premier experts in genital herpes.*

Corey L, Wald A. Maternal and neonatal herpes simplex virus infections. *N Engl J Med.* 2009;361:1376-85. *Review of clinical manifestations, perinatal transmission, and management of herpes in pregnant women and newborns, and strategies to prevent neonatal herpes.*

Mark KE, et al. Rapidly cleared episodes of herpes simplex virus reactivation in immunocompetent adults. *J Infect Dis.* 2008;198:1141-9. *Documentation of frequent, brief episodes of subclinical viral shedding in most HSV infected persons and an introduction to the concept of genital and oral herpes as continuously active rather than episodic infections.*

Mertz K, et al. Etiology of genital ulcers and prevalence of human immunodeficiency virus coinfection in 10 US cities. *J Infect Dis.* 1998;178:1975-8. *A large observational study of patients presenting with genital ulcer disease, using PCR for HSV,* T. pallidum, *and* Haemophilis ducreyi, *documenting herpes as the cause of over 60%, despite selection of clinics with high rates of syphilis or chancroid.*

Tobian AA, Quinn TC. Herpes simplex virus type 2 and syphilis infections with HIV: an evolving synergy in transmission and prevention. *Curr Opin HIV AIDS.* 2009;4:294-9. *A concise review emphasizing the role of HSV-2, as well as syphilis, in promoting sexual transmission of HIV.*

9

Human Papillomavirus Infection and Genital Warts

Anogenital infection with human papillomavirus (HPV), long considered an inconvenient but benign condition, has emerged as one of the most important as well as one of the most common STDs. HPV is ubiquitous, and at least 80% of sexually active persons acquire at least one anogenital infection during their sexually active lives. Reflecting both high prevalence and efficient sexual transmission, up to half of all persons are infected within their first three lifetime sex partners, and the prevalence of genital HPV ranges from 20 to 50% in most sexually active populations. Over 100 HPV types are known, of which about 40 usually infect the genital tract or anus and are transmitted primarily if not exclusively by sexual contact. Anogenital HPV strains comprise two broad classes, based on their association with cancer and premalignant neoplasia. "Low-risk" HPV types are infrequently implicated in cancer or high-grade dysplasia, although they often cause low-grade dysplasia that regresses without treatment. Among the low-risk types are HPV-6 and 11, which cause 85 to 90% of anogenital warts. "High-risk" HPV types, such as HPV-16, 18, 31, 45, and several others, cause dysplasia and cancer of the cervix, anus, penis, and vulva. HPV-16 and 18 account for 65 to 70% of cervical cancers and precancerous dysplasia, with remarkably similar prevalences in all populations worldwide; there is somewhat greater variation in the frequencies of other oncogenic types like HPV-31, 45, and others. Among asymptomatic persons tested for genital HPV infection, HPV-16 is the most common type overall in both the general population and those at high risk for STD. The type distributions are similar in both sexes and for vaginal, penile, and anal HPV infections.

Anogenital HPV-6 and 11 infections result in overt warts in about two-thirds of infected persons, but most other anogenital HPV infections remain subclinical, causing neither symptoms nor dysplasia. Although HPV DNA may persist for life in squamous epithelium, detectable infection using currently available technologies usually resolves spontaneously within 6–12 months for low-risk HPV types and 12–24 months for HPV-16 and 18. However, late recurrence is not rare and accounts for some genital warts and probably most cases of dysplasia or cancer in persons

≥30 years old. Reinfection with the same HPV type appears to be infrequent, probably owing to acquired immunity. Because no treatment has been shown to eliminate the virus from infected skin and mucous membranes, the primary goals for clinical management are elimination of symptomatic warts, treatment of malignancy and premalignant changes, and counseling to limit psychosocial distress.

For half a century, prevention of HPV morbidity in industrialized countries has been based primarily on cervical cytology to detect and treat dysplasia and carcinoma in situ. Since 1960, annual rates of cervical cancer in the United States and most industrialized countries have declined from 30 to 40 cases to 8 to 10 cases per 100,000 women. Cytology-based prevention is beyond the means of most developing countries, but detection of high-risk HPV by nucleic acid amplification tests (NAATs) (e.g., using self-collected vaginal swabs) now has promise for cervical cancer prevention. Most important, the means are now at hand for primary prevention of anogenital HPV infection through immunization. The development of effective vaccines against selected HPV types—biologically among the most effective vaccines ever produced—was a milestone in both STD prevention and cancer prevention. Bivalent (HPV-16 and 18) and quadrivalent (HPV-6, 11, 16, and 18) vaccines are currently available, and vaccines with expanded strain coverage are in development. Routine immunization is now recommended for all young women and girls. Because risk for HPV begins immediately after onset of sexual activity and incident infections are common in sexually active teens, maximum benefit from immunization requires vaccination of girls prior to sexual debut, ideally before age 12. Immunization of boys and men also is increasingly advised, both to limit HPV morbidity in men, especially anal cancer, and to help prevent transmission of HPV to women. Condoms significantly reduce the risk of anogenital HPV infection but protection is incomplete, and all prevention strategies other than immunization have limited efficacy, partly because multiple anogenital HPV strains remain ubiquitous and efficiently transmitted.

Oral infections with genital HPV types are not uncommon, but most are subclinical. The rates of tonsilar and other posterior pharyngeal cancers associated with HPV-16 are rising in the United States and perhaps elsewhere, perhaps the result of rising frequencies of orogenital sex in recent decades. However, these malignancies remain rare, and many cases continue to occur in persons >50 years old with other risk factors like tobacco and alcohol abuse. Even if HPV-16 is the direct cause of these malignancies, the link to sexual acquisition of oral HPV infection is tenuous, and it remains to be seen whether immunization will protect against HPV-16-related pharyngeal cancer. Research is evolving rapidly and clinicians should be alert to new developments and improved understanding of oral HPV infection and its consequences.

This chapter primarily addresses the epidemiologic and clinical aspects of anogenital warts. Other sources should be consulted for diagnosis and management of HPV-related malignancies and premalignant lesions, including management of women with abnormal cervical cytology.

EPIDEMIOLOGY

Incidence and Prevalence

- Estimated incidence 6 million anogenital HPV infections annually in the United States

- In most countries, >80% of sexually active persons acquire one or more genital HPV infections

- Prevalence 20–50% in most sexually active populations age 15–40 years in the United States

- In the United States, 6% of all persons (males 4%, females 7%) report past history of genital warts, including 11% of persons with ≥10 lifetime sex partners; genital warts account for 300,000–400,000 physician visits per year

- Population-based modeling studies in Scandinavia suggest lifetime risk of genital warts approximates 15–20%

- Overall rates are similar in most populations worldwide

- Anogenital HPV is almost equally prevalent in populations at low and high risk for other STDs

Transmission

- Sexual contact, probably enhanced by friction or microtrauma
  - Most cases transmitted by vaginal or anal intercourse
  - Genital to oral transmission may be frequent, but symptomatic oral HPV is uncommon
  - Oral to genital transmission probably is uncommon
  - Transmission by hand-genital contact, directly or by exchange of genital secretions, probably is uncommon, but may explain some cases in infected persons who deny other sexual exposures

- Autoinoculation to nongenital sites may occur, but clinical manifestations are rare at sites other than genitals or anus

- Perinatal transmission to newborns during vaginal delivery can cause respiratory papillomatosis; infrequent but potentially serious

- Fomite transmission occurs rarely if ever

Age

- Most infections acquired by persons from age of sexual debut to 30 years old

Sex

- No specific predilection known for HPV infection per se

- More frequently diagnosed in women than men due to Pap screening and more frequent attendance for health care

Sexual Orientation

- No predilection for HPV infection per se

- Anogenital infection with both high- and low-risk HPV is common in both MSM and WSW

- Among MSM, annual anal cancer rate approximates 35–40 per 100,000 (equivalent to cervical cancer rate in absence of routine Pap smears)

Other Risk Factors

- Circumcision in men is partly protective; warts and subclinical penile HPV infection are less frequent in circumcised than uncircumcised men

- Cellular immunodeficiency (e.g., advanced HIV infection) is associated with recrudescence of warts, atypical locations (e.g., oral and facial), and probably accelerated progression of dysplasia and cancer

HISTORY

Incubation Period

- Exophytic warts typically appear 2–12 months after exposure (mean 6–8 months)
- Cervical dysplasia can develop within several weeks of acquiring HPV; severe dysplasia and, rarely, carcinoma in situ can develop without intervening mild dysplasia
- Progression to invasive cancer typically requires 5–30 years, but can occur within 1 year

Symptoms

- High-risk HPV infections usually are asymptomatic
- Anogenital warts are the most common symptom; 60–70% of HPV-6 or 11 infections result in overt warts
- HPV infection per se rarely if ever causes pruritus, burning, or similar symptoms (notwithstanding common perceptions by some patients)
- Large or traumatized warts may ulcerate or become secondarily infected, with itching, pain, discharge, or malodor
- Urethral warts in men may cause altered urine stream and, rarely, outflow obstruction
- External genital or anal neoplastic lesions, such as vulvar intraepithelial neoplasia (VIN), and comparable lesions of the vagina (VaIN), penis (PIN), or anus (AIN)
- Respiratory papillomatosis in infants, and rarely in adults, can cause hoarseness and, in advanced cases, airway obstruction

Epidemiologic History

- Most patients with new anogenital warts acknowledge new sexual partnerships in preceding 1–2 years
- Many persons with subclinical HPV infection lack recent behavioral STD risks

PHYSICAL EXAMINATION

- Genital wart morphology
  - Condylomata acuminata (singular, condyloma acuminatum): Moist or partially keratinized surfaces (e.g., introitus, anus, under foreskin); typical "cauliflower" appearance; central venules in fronds may be observed with handheld magnification or colposcopy
  - Keratotic warts: Horny, often cauliflower-like appearance, typically on dry skin, e.g., penile shaft, scrotum, labia majora
  - Papular warts: Smooth surface, less horny than keratotic warts
  - Flat warts: Macular or faintly raised; usually invisible to naked eye
- Anatomic sites are primarily those most subject to friction during sex
  - Penile glans or shaft, especially under foreskin of uncircumcised men
  - Vaginal introitus, labia minora
  - Anus: Anal warts most commonly observed in MSM, acquired by receptive anal sex; also frequent in women (with or without anal sex); less frequently but nevertheless common in heterosexual men (probably by autoinoculation or contiguous spread)

- ○ Urethral, vaginal, cervical, or rectal mucosa

- ○ Perigenital areas such as scrotum, labia majora, or groin are less frequently involved, but not rare

- Visual inspection in good light, sometimes aided by magnification, usually is sufficient for accurate diagnosis of anogenital warts

- Recognition or suspicion of other HPV-related anogenital lesions, such as overt anogenital cancer, Bowenoid papulosis, VIN, PIN, AIN, or VaIN, requires considerable expertise and confirmation by biopsy

- Application of 3% acetic acid may highlight HPV-infected skin or mucosa ("acetowhitening") to identify subclinical infection, but both false-positive and false-negative results are common; not recommended except by well-trained experts

- Colposcopy is routine in evaluation of women with cervical dysplasia or other Pap smear abnormalities and can identify cervical or vaginal warts

- Anoscopy may reveal rectal warts, but importance of detecting or treating asymptomatic rectal warts is unknown

- Screen patients with newly diagnosed anogenital warts or abnormal cytology for other common STDs and HIV

LABORATORY DIAGNOSIS

Cytology, especially of the cervix and increasingly on anal specimens, is time-honored and remains the primary method to identify presumed HPV infections of mucosal surfaces, especially the cervix. Nucleic acid amplification tests (NAATs) are available to detect HPV, typically classified as high or low risk (usually without determination of individual HPV types), to guide management of patients with abnormal Pap smears, and may have an independent role in screening to identify persons at risk for cervical or anal cancer where Pap smears are not readily available, especially in developing countries. Currently available HPV NAATs are neither approved nor recommended to diagnose asymptomatic HPV infection in males or for anatomic sites other than the cervix, vagina, and anus.

- Typical changes on cervical cytology (Pap smear):
  - ○ High-grade and low-grade squamous intraepithelial lesions (HSIL and LSIL, respectively) and carcinoma in situ always indicate HPV infection
  - ○ HPV is present in about half of patients with atypical squamous or glandular cells of undetermined significance (ASCUS, AGUS)

- HPV NAAT can help guide management of patients with selected cytologic abnormalities, e.g., observation and repeat Pap smear versus early colposcopy and biopsy; may supplant Pap smear in some settings (research in progress)

- Screening MSM for anal dysplasia and cancer with anal cytology and/or HPV NAAT is advocated by some investigators but not currently recommended for routine use

- Type-specific HPV antibody tests are used for research but currently have insufficient performance for reliable clinical use

DIFFERENTIAL DIAGNOSIS OF ANOGENITAL WARTS

Visual diagnosis is adequate for most exophytic warts, but biopsy is indicated for pigmented and other atypical lesions, those that do not respond to treatment or have clinical appearances suggestive of malignancy or premalignant changes, such as Bowenoid papulosis, leukoplakia, and penile, vulvar, vaginal, and anal intraepithelial neoplasia (PIN, VIN, VaIN, and AIN, respectively) and overt squamous cell cancers. Pathologic and normal findings commonly mistaken for anogenital warts include molluscum contagiosum (see Chap 10), condylomata lata of syphilis (see Chap. 5), pearly penile papules, skin tags, Tyson glands, and other anatomic variants (see Chap. 22).

TREATMENT OF ANOGENITAL WARTS

Principles

The primary goal of treatment is to eradicate overt warts; no available therapy has been shown to eradicate HPV. Eliminating visible warts might reduce the risk of sexual transmission, but no data are available. Surgical excision, laser cautery, or electrocautery immediately ablate visible warts. Other modalities (cryotherapy, podophyllin, podofilox, sinecatechins, tri- or bichloroacetic acid, imiquimod) have 60–80% efficacy within several weeks, but the therapeutic response is highly variable from one patient to another. Recurrence of warts within 2–3 months is equally common with all therapies. Combination methods, such as cryotherapy plus podophyllin, speeds resolution in some patients. When therapy is unsuccessful or in event of prompt recurrence, an alternate method should be used. Other factors that influence choice of treatment include size and number of warts, anatomic site, provider experience, cutaneous versus mucosal surfaces, cost, and preference for patient-applied or provider-applied treatment. Treatment is not recommended for subclinical anogenital or oral infection that may be diagnosed by colposcopy, application of acetic acid to normal-appearing skin or mucosa, or positive NAAT for HPV.

Patient-Applied Treatment of External Warts

Podofilox (Condylox) is a purified antimitotic agent derived from podophyllin, chemically related to the vinca alkaloids. Sinechatechins (Veregen) is a green tea extract that has been effective against genital warts in uncontrolled clinical trials. Imiquimod (Aldara) is an immune enhancer that stimulates local production of interferon and other cytokines, a mechanism that might be especially effective in preventing recurrent warts. However, a reduced recurrence rate has not been documented for imiquimod, response of warts typically is slower than with other patient-applied treatments, and efficacy is reduced for lesions on dry compared with moist surfaces. Safety in pregnancy is unknown for all of the recommended patient-applied regimens.

- Podofilox 0.5% solution or gel: apply to warts *bid* for 3 days, followed by 4 treatment-free days; repeat weekly up to 4 cycles

- Imiquimod 5% cream: apply to warts once daily at bedtime and wash off after 6–10 hours; repeat 3 times weekly for up to 16 weeks

- Sinecatechins 15% ointment: apply to warts *tid* until warts resolved; maximum 16 weeks

Provider-Applied Therapy of External Warts

Selection of provider-applied treatments is primarily determined by availability in particular clinical settings and provider experience, and secondarily by cost, desire for immediate ablation of warts, size of warts, and anatomic location. Cryotherapy destroys wart tissue by thermal cellular disruption. Podophyllin resin is an antimitotic agent that is selectively toxic for neoplastic tissues, including warts. Podophyllin preparations are not well standardized and may have variable efficacy; concentrations of 10–25% are available. Trichloroacetic acid and bichloroacetic acid are caustic agents that coagulate and destroy tissue proteins.

- Cryotherapy with liquid nitrogen or cryoprobe: repeat weekly until warts resolved; 2–4 treatments usually required; main side effects are local irritation and ulceration

- Podophyllin resin, 10–25% in tincture of benzoin
  - Apply to warts, minimizing contact with uninvolved tissue; allow to air dry
  - Wash to remove resin 1 hour after application (optional; may reduce local irritation)
  - Maximum dose 0.5 mL or 10 cm^2 of treated tissue (to minimize systemic absorption)
  - Repeat weekly as needed; several treatments usually required
  - Primary side effects are local irritation and ulceration
  - Contraindicated in pregnancy

- Trichloroacetic acid or bichloroacetic acid, 80–90% solution
  - Apply to warts, with care to avoid contact with uninvolved tissue
  - Repeat weekly as needed
  - Several treatments usually required
  - Local irritation and ulceration are primary side effects

- Surgical removal by scissor excision, tangential shave excision, electrocautery, laser cautery, etc. (special training required)

- Alternative regimens include intralesional interferon, photodynamic therapy, topical cidofovir, and isotretinoin; generally less effective, poorly studied, and expensive

Treatment of Mucosal Warts

Podophyllin, podofilox, imiquimod, and sinecatechins are not recommended for use on most mucosal surfaces, except that podophyllin resin can be used to treat vaginal warts. Options for vaginal, urethral, anal, rectal, and oral warts include cryotherapy, tri- or bichloroacetic acid, or surgical excision. Surgical removal is the main treatment for cervical warts or precancerous dysplasia.

Follow-up

- Routine follow-up not indicated after visible warts resolved

- Reevaluate if warts persist or recur

Partner Management

- Partners with symptoms (e.g., suspected warts) should be evaluated; advise patients that incubation period for visible warts may be up to 2 years.
- Routine referral and examination are not indicated for asymptomatic partners of patients with anogenital warts, abnormal cervical cytology, or other evidence of HPV infection
  - Partners with ongoing exposure to infected patients can be assumed to be infected
  - No recommended diagnostic tests are available
  - No treatment is available for subclinical infection
- Prospective (future) partners may be offered HPV immunization

PREVENTION AND COUNSELING

- Ablation of warts and treatment of cervical or anal dysplasia may reduce viral load and perhaps transmission risk, but no data are available
- Transmission risk probably is low after warts or dysplasia are successfully treated and do not recur 3-6 months after treatment
- Most HPV infections are subclinical and remain so
- Cancer and other serious complications are uncommon
- Anogenital warts and cancers are caused by different HPV types
- HPV is readily transmissible by genital and perhaps orogenital exposure
- All sexually active persons can expect to have one or more anogenital HPV infections, usually without symptoms or serious medical consequences
- Most infections resolve spontaneously, with or without treatment
- Condoms reduce risk of infection or transmission, but protection is incomplete; substantial likelihood of HIV infection persists in consistent condom users
- Partners who have been sexually active with the index patient prior to diagnosis should assume they are infected; they should be on the lookout for warts and other symptoms; no treatment or evaluation is indicated in absence of clinical manifestations
- HPV immunization is recommended for sexually active persons $\leq$26 years old, including those with clinical manifestations of HPV (e.g., genital warts, abnormal Pap smear)

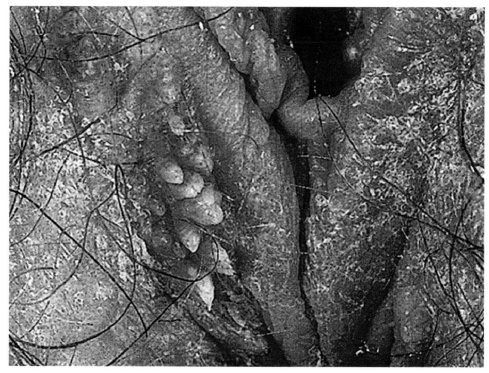

9–1. Genital warts of labia majora and perineum, with features of both condylomata acuminata and keratotic warts.

CASE

Patient Profile Age 23, single graduate student

History Painless genital "bumps" for 1 month; monogamous in a relationship that began 4 months earlier

Examination "Cauliflower-like" excrescences, some with horny surface, of labia majora and perineum

Diagnosis Genital warts (condylomata acuminata and keratotic warts)

Laboratory Routine screening for other STDs, including serological tests for syphilis and HIV, cervical NAATs for *C. trachomatis* and *N. gonorrhoeae*; Pap smear done 4 months earlier, not repeated

Treatment Cryotherapy with liquid nitrogen; repeat treatments scheduled weekly until resolved

Partner Management Patient was advised to refer partner if he noticed genital warts or other lesions, otherwise no need for examination

Comment The patient expressed concern about cancer risk and was counseled that warts and cervical and other cancers are caused by separate HPV types. She was advised to continue routine Pap smears as directed by her reproductive health provider, and to report persisting or recurrent external genital lesions. She was further advised that most HPV infections eventually resolve (with or without treatment) and that late recurrence is possible but uncommon.

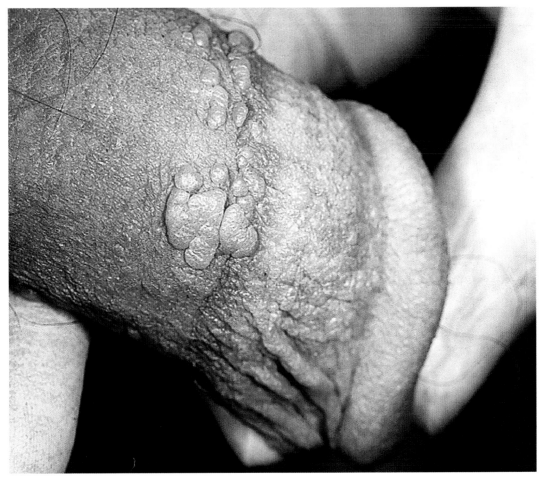

9–2. Multiple condylomatous and papular penile warts.

CASE

Patient Profile Age 26, single bookstore manager

History Painless penile growths for 6 weeks; 3 sex partners in past year

Examination Several 1- to 5-mm excrescences of penile shaft, some appearing "cauliflower-like," others smooth

Laboratory Screening tests for syphilis, gonorrhea, chlamydial infection, and HIV (all negative)

Diagnosis Genital warts (condylomata acuminata and papular warts)

Treatment Cryotherapy with liquid nitrogen, followed by self-treatment with podofilox gel 0.5% for up to 4 weeks

Comment The patient was about to move to another city and requested continued self-applied therapy instead of returning for repeat cryotherapy. He was advised to inform partners of his diagnosis, who should seek examination if warts become apparent.

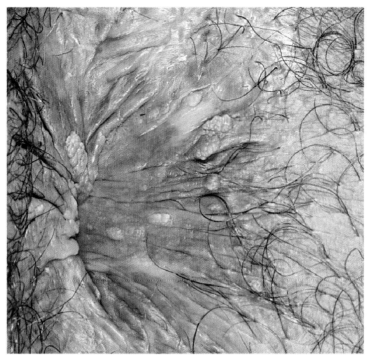

9–3. Anal warts (condylomata acuminata).

CASE

Patient Profile Age 43, HIV-infected male television cameraman

History Anal "bumps" and itching for 1 week; history of anal warts that resolved after treatment with podophyllin 6 years earlier; monogamous with male partner for 2 years, denied receptive anal intercourse in past few months; HIV infection diagnosed 2 years earlier, with intermittent medical follow-up (not taking antiretroviral therapy); denied fever, weight loss, or other systemic symptoms

Examination Numerous anal and perianal excrescences with predominantly "cauliflower-like" morphology; anoscopy normal, without visible mucosal warts; general physical examination normal

Differential Diagnosis Anal warts; rule out anal cancer and syphilis (condylomata lata)

Laboratory Syphilis serology (negative); rectal cultures for *N. gonorrhoeae* and *C. trachomatis* negative

Diagnosis Anal condylomata acuminata; HIV infection

Treatment Cryotherapy with liquid nitrogen, repeated weekly

Comment The patient was referred to a proctologist for reassessment of intrarectal lesions and for consideration of biopsy to exclude anal dysplasia and cancer. He was advised that reappearance of warts might suggest progression of immunodeficiency and was referred to a local HIV/AIDS clinic to resume regular health care for HIV infection.

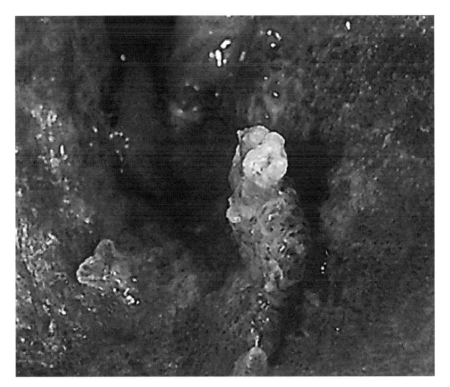

9–4. Condylomata acuminata of the vaginal introitus, with keratotic changes at the terminus of the largest wart. Central venules can be seen in individual fronds.

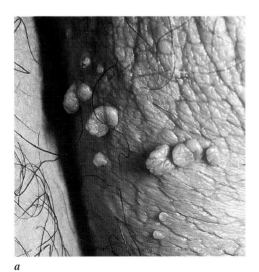

a

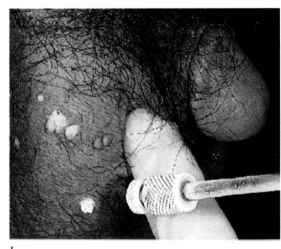

b

9–5. Genital warts of scrotum. *a*. Condylomata acuminata and papular warts. *b*. Cryotherapy with liquid nitrogen.

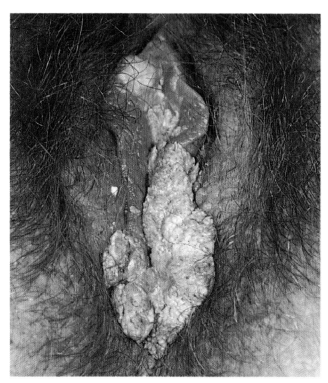

9–6. Giant warts (Buschke-Löwenstein tumor) of vulva. Malignant changes sometimes occur, and such lesions should be biopsied. Secondary infection and infarction necrosis are common complications.

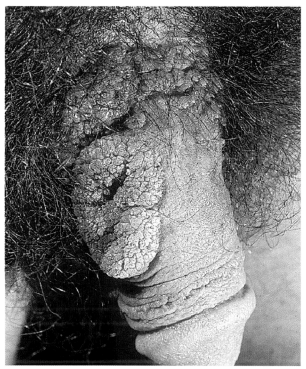

9–7. Neglected penile warts progressing to giant condylomata.

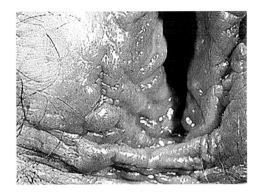

9–8. Papular warts of vaginal introitus and perineum.

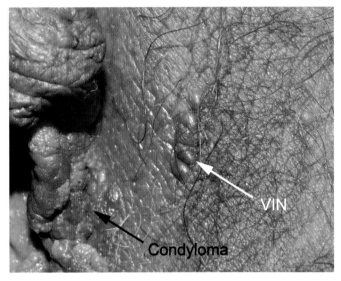

9–9. Nodular pigmented lesions of vulvar intraepithelial neoplasia (VIN) (white arrow). The patient also has benign condylomata acuminata (black arrow). (*Courtesy of Hope Haefner, M.D.*)

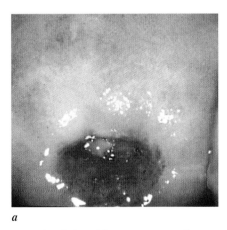

a

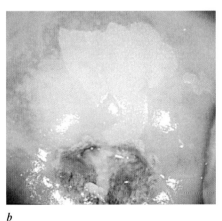

b

9–10. Cervix with subclinical flat wart. *a.* Normal-appearing ectocervix. *b.* Flat wart revealed by application of 3% acetic acid, viewed in green light. Note that flat wart does not coincide with the area of relative pallor observed before acetic acid application. Mucopurulent exudate is present in cervical os; *C. trachomatis* was isolated. (*Courtesy of Claire E. Stevens.*)

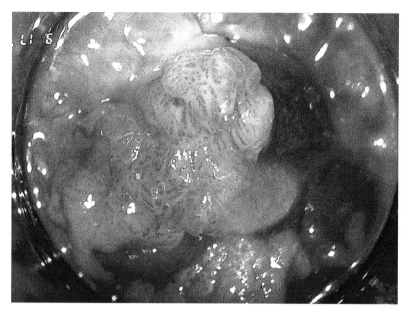

9–11. Large condylomata acuminata of rectal mucosa, viewed by anoscopy. (*Courtesy of Christina M. Surawicz, M.D.*)

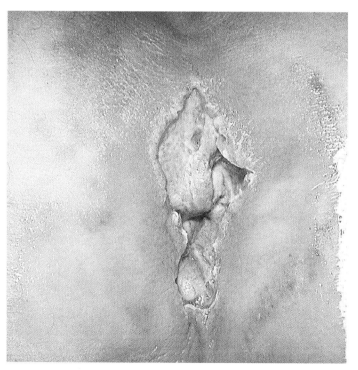

9–12. Invasive HPV-related squamous cell cancer of the anus in a man with AIDS. (*Courtesy of Steven J. Medwell, M.D.*)

SUGGESTED READING

Fairley CK, et al. Rapid decline in presentations of genital warts after the implementation of a national quadrivalent human papillomavirus vaccination programme for young women. *Sex Transm Infect.* 2009;85:499-502. *An ecological study documenting public health benefit through herd immunity, manifested by reduced frequency of genital warts in men as well as women.*

Garland SM, Smith JS. Human papillomavirus vaccines: current status and future prospects. *Drugs.* 2010;70:1079-98. *Comprehensive literature review of the efficacy, indications, utility, and public health impact of the currently available HPV vaccines.*

Kennedy CM, Boardman LA. New approaches to external genital warts and vulvar intraepithelial neoplasia. *Clin Obstet Gynecol.* 2008;51:518-26. *A review of clinical manifestations, diagnosis, and treatment of external genital HPV disease in women.*

Palefsky JM. Human papillomavirus-related disease in men: not just a women's issue. *J Adolesc Health.* 2010;46(4 Suppl):S12-9. *A useful review of epidemiology and clinical aspects of HPV-related diseases in men, including penile and anal cancer.*

Pirotta M, et al. The psychological burden of human papillomavirus related disease and screening interventions. *Sex Transm Infect.* 2009;85:508-13. *A prospective study documenting substantial emotional impact when genital warts or other HPV infections are diagnosed.*

Winer RL, et al. Risk of female human papillomavirus acquisition associated with first male sex partner. *J Infect Dis.* 2008;197:279-82. *A prospective study showing a 28% one year cumulative incidence of first HPV infection in young women with only one lifetime male sex partner; risk of infection was associated with male partners' sexual experience.*

Winer RL, Koutsky LA. Genital human papillomavirus infection. Chapter 28 in KK Holmes, et al., eds. *Sexually Transmitted Diseases.* 4th ed.. New York, NY: McGraw-Hill 2008:489-508. *A comprehensive introduction to HPV and genital warts by leading investigators, in the premier STD textbook.*

10

Molluscum Contagiosum

Molluscum contagiosum is a common cutaneous viral eruption that on cursory inspection may resemble warts. The molluscum contagiosum virus (MCV) is a pox virus; two types (MCV-1, MCV-2) have been described. The virus has not been cultivated, because only mature keratinocytes are susceptible and such cells have not been successfully propagated. The infection most commonly involves the face and upper extremities in young children, who are infected by contact with saliva of other children, typically in nursery or school settings. Genital area infection usually is sexually acquired and is common in sexually active teens and young adults, and probably occurs primarily in those who escaped childhood infection and lack protective immunity. In sexually active adults, molluscum usually involves the pubic area, lower abdomen, upper thighs, or buttocks, as well as external genitals. Facial lesions can occur in imunodeficient adults, such as persons with AIDS, probably the result of reactivation of latent infection when immune surveillance wanes. With few exceptions, molluscum contagiosum is a benign condition with few complications except for cosmetic effects and the psychological impact of a sexually transmitted disease (STD). Treatment is effective with any of several destructive methods, and most cases resolve within a few months without therapy.

EPIDEMIOLOGY

Incidence and Prevalence

- No reliable statistics available
- Rising frequency has been reported in some STD clinics in recent years

Transmission

- Sexual or salivary transmission
- Autoinoculation probably accounts for some cases of regional spread of lesions, e.g. by pubic shaving

Age

- Most cases occur in young children
- In sexually active adults, most common age is 15–30 years

Sex

- No known predisposition

Sexual Orientation

- No known predisposition

Other Risk Factors

- Cellular immunodeficiency risks late recrudescence; facial lesions can be a difficult management problem in patients with AIDS

HISTORY

Incubation Period

- Usually 2–3 months, range 1 week to 6 months

Symptoms

- Painless papules or wart-like bumps, often with a shiny pink appearance and central depression
- Sexually acquired lesions are located primarily in genital and perigenital areas, e.g., lower abdomen, pubic area, upper thighs
- May be asymptomatic or unrecognized

Epidemiologic History

- Behavioral risks for STD
- Sometimes sexual contact with known case

PHYSICAL EXAMINATION

- In immunocompetent persons, usually several smooth, waxy, erythematous papules, often with central umbilication
- Most common on penis or labia, and perigenital locations (pubic area, upper thighs, scrotum, etc.)
- Facial, scalp, and other sites are common in children and persons with AIDS

DIAGNOSIS

- Usually diagnosed by clinical appearance
- May be confused with genital warts
- Examine small lesions under magnification
- Expression of hard, white core, followed by brisk bleeding confirms diagnosis
- Characteristic histopathology if lesions are biopsied
- Screen for other STDs

TREATMENT

- Few controlled trials reported, only in young children; recommendations in adults are based on uncontrolled observational reports
- Freezing by liquid nitrogen or cryoprobe
- Curettage
- Imiquimod 5% cream 3–5 times per week for up to 16 weeks
- If few in number, lesions may be unroofed with needle and core manually expressed, although this may carry risk of local autoinoculation
- Podofilox, cantharadin, and other chemical irritants have been reported to be effective

SEX PARTNER MANAGEMENT

- Counsel patients to advise partners to seek treatment if lesions noted

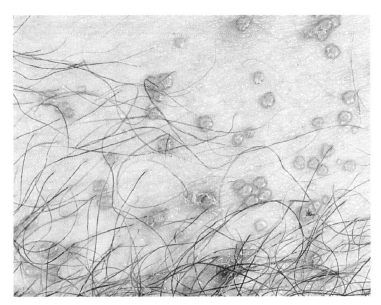

10–1. Multiple lesions of molluscum contagiosum on lower abdomen. Individual lesions do not have emanating hairs or surrounding erythema, excluding folliculitis (see Fig. 22-14). Central umbilication, pink color, shiny appearance, and multiple lesions with little variation in size and morphology distinguish molluscum from genital warts.

CASE

Patient Profile Age 19, male college sophomore

History Painless pink growths on lower abdomen and pubic area, first noted 2 weeks earlier; sexually active with new girlfriend for 2 months

Examination Numerous 1- to 3-mm smooth, erythematous, waxy papules, most with central umbilication; individual lesions not associated with hairs

Differential Diagnosis Molluscum contagiosum, genital warts, syphilis (condylomata lata), other papular eruptions; one lesion was unroofed with a needle and white core expressed, followed by brisk bleeding

Laboratory Screening tests for chlamydial infection, gonorrhea, syphilis, and HIV

Diagnosis Molluscum contagiosum

Treatment Cryotherapy with liquid nitrogen, repeated in 1 week

Partner Management Advised to refer girlfriend if she notes lesions

Comment The lesions largely resolved following cryotherapy, but 2 weeks later several new lesions had appeared, a typical clinical course. The patient was prescribed imiquimod for self-treatment for subsequent lesions and advised that he should expect new lesions to stop appearing within 1–2 months.

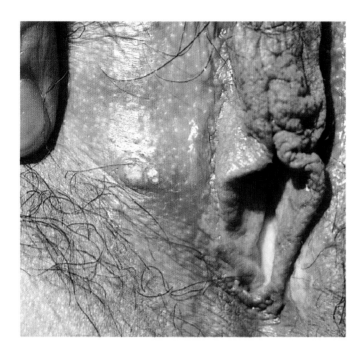

10–2. Atypical molluscum contagiosum, with loss of superficial epithelium and presenting as a nodular vulvar ulcer. Patient also has discharge due to bacterial vaginosis (see Fig. 19–3).

CASE

Patient Profile Age 20, single, enlisted woman in U.S. Army

History Painless vulvar "bump" for 1 week; malodorous vaginal discharge intermittently for an undetermined period; monogamous for past year, but boyfriend suspected to have other partners

Examination Nontender, nodular, ulcerated lesion of vulva with firm, white base; homogeneous, white vaginal discharge

Differential Diagnosis Syphilis, genital wart, herpes, chancroid, molluscum contagiosum, granuloma inguinale, cancer

Laboratory Darkfield examination, VDRL, culture for HSV, and screening tests for *N. gonorrhoeae* and *C. trachomatis* (all negative); referred to dermatologist for biopsy; on attempt at punch biopsy, a hard white core was expressed; molluscum contagiosum was confirmed histologically; pH 5.0, amine odor test positive, clue cells seen microscopically

Diagnosis Molluscum contagiosum; bacterial vaginosis

Treatment Cryotherapy with liquid nitrogen; metronidazole 500 mg PO *bid* for 7 days

Partner Management Advised to refer partner for STD screening

Comment In this atypical case, the patient presented with ulcerated molluscum contagiosum, a rarely recognized clinical entity. Partner evaluation for molluscum is recommended only when lesions are noted by partners, but the patient's bacterial vaginosis and sexual history suggested value in STD screening of the partner. However, he did not attend the clinic and the patient was lost to follow-up.

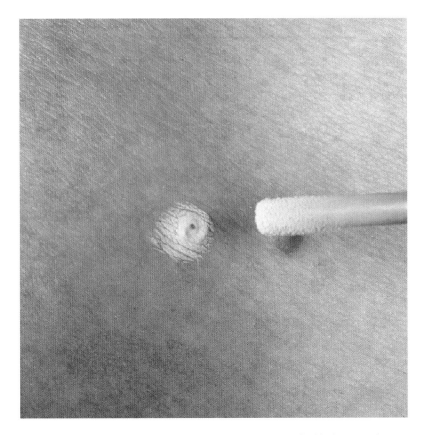

10–3. Molluscum contagiosum. Freezing with liquid nitrogen highlights central umbilication.

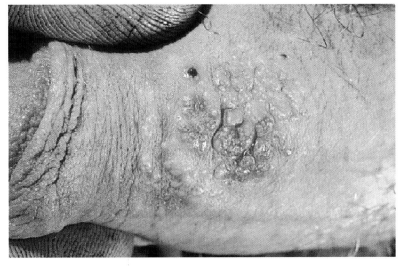

10–4. Molluscum contagiosum; confluent lesions of penis. Note bleeding after expression of the core of a lesion.

SUGGESTED READING

Douglas JM, Jr. Molluscum contagiosum. Chapter 30 in KK Holmes, et al., eds. *Sexually Transmitted Diseases*. 4th ed. New York, NY: McGraw-Hill; 2008:545-52. *A concise, up-to-date review in the premier STD textbook.*

Villa L, et al. Molluscum contagiosum: a 20-year study in a sexually transmitted infections unit. *Sex Transm Dis*. 2010;37:423-4. *Documentation of a substantial rise in frequency of molluscum contagiosum in an STD clinic from 1988 through 2008.*

11

Human Immunodeficiency Virus Infection

The acquired immunodeficiency syndrome (AIDS) is by far the most important STD of all time, responsible for substantially more morbidity and loss of life than syphilis in its heyday. The causative agents, human immunodeficiency virus (HIV) types 1 and 2, are transmitted by intimate exposure to blood as well as to sexual and certain other body secretions, and sexual activity is the main transmission route worldwide. HIV-1 is the predominant virus type worldwide and is responsible for almost all infections diagnosed in the United States and most industrialized countries. To date HIV-2 infections are limited to endemic areas and a few cases imported from those areas.

Particular sexual practices have variable HIV transmission efficiencies. Vaginal intercourse is the dominant route of transmission globally, but not the most efficient mode. Sexual transmission efficiency is highest by anal intercourse, largely explaining the high rates of HIV/AIDS in men who have sex with men (MSM). Transmission by blood exchange through illicit drug use, with shared injection equipment, contributes variably to HIV transmission in different populations. Mother-to-child transmission of HIV during labor and delivery and postnatally through nursing explains most infections in young children. Nosocomial transmission to health workers, primarily though injury with contaminated sharp instruments, is inefficient and infrequent. Transmission by transfusion and organ transplantation now is rare worldwide, owing to routine, universal testing of donors. Universal testing of pregnant women, combined with antiretroviral (ARV) therapy of infants born to infected mothers, has greatly curtailed perinatal transmission in industrialized countries and is beginning to have substantial impact in many developing countries.

All inflammatory STDs are associated with enhanced efficiency of HIV acquisition in exposed persons, increased transmission of HIV by dually infected individuals, or both. Noninflammatory STDs like bacterial vaginosis and human papillomavirus infection also may increase HIV transmission risk. Owing to the high prevalence of infection with herpes simplex virus type 2 (HSV-2) in most populations, HSV-2 has the greatest population-level influence of all STDs on HIV transmission, and in some populations up to half of all HIV transmission events may be attributable to HSV-2. HSV-1 infection, whether oral or genital, apparently has little if any influence on HIV risk. These associations imply that treatment of STDs might blunt the spread of HIV, but that concept has been difficult to prove. In large randomized controlled trials, suppressive treatment of HSV-2 infected persons with acyclovir did not reduce the incidence of HIV and, with one exception, several trials of treatment for bacterial STDs had no demonstrable effect on HIV transmission. Nonetheless, HIV shedding and susceptibility clearly are enhanced by many STDs, and HIV viral load in genital secretions falls dramatically following treatment of gonorrhea, genital herpes, and other STDs. Notwithstanding the clinical trial results, it remains likely that treatment of STD does indeed reduce individual patients' risk of acquiring or transmitting HIV, and successful prevention of STDs probably helps limit the spread of HIV.

Male circumcision also is an important factor in heterosexual transmission of HIV, and three large randomized controlled trials in southern Africa documented about a 50% reduction in incident HIV infections following circumcision of sexually active adult men. However, the fraction of HIV infections attributable to circumcision status is highly variable in different populations, and the importance of either adult or routine infant circumcision for HIV prevention in industrialized countries is unknown. Behavioral factors that operate at both individual and population levels, such as number of sex partners and especially rates of concurrency (overlapping partnerships) in sex partner networks, are among the most important determinants of HIV spread (see Chap. 1). Wide variations in these factors, combined with differences in STD rates and the frequency of routine male circumcision, are the primary reasons for the widely divergent rates of heterosexually transmitted HIV infection between countries, regions, and populations.

Clinicians who provide STD care should be prepared to recognize the common signs and symptoms of HIV infection and AIDS, and should provide serological screening and diagnostic testing for HIV infection. Routine HIV screening, with opt-out consent and without required pre-test risk assessment or counseling, is recommended in the United States by the Centers for Disease Control and Prevention (CDC) for all 13- to 64-year-old persons obtaining health care for any reason, and similar strategies likely would bring enhanced prevention benefits in most countries. All clinicians providing STD services should be prepared to provide postexposure prophylaxis with antiretroviral drugs when patients present following exposures with high risk of HIV transmission, and to either provide comprehensive management for HIV infected persons or to have an established referral plan for their infected patients. It is beyond the scope of this book to review all aspects of HIV infection or to address the increasingly complex therapeutic aspects of HIV/AIDS and opportunistic diseases. Rather, the focus is on the epidemiology of HIV infection, prevention, and the recognition of HIV infection and AIDS. The emphasis is on the United States, but the information is applicable to most industrialized countries. Selected aspects pertinent to developing countries are addressed in Chap. 2.

EPIDEMIOLOGY

Incidence and Prevalence

- Incidence in the United States estimated 56,300 HIV infections per year in 2006
- Prevalence in the United States estimated 1.1 million persons living with HIV at end of 2007
- Through 2007, about 576,000 U.S. residents had died of AIDS
- Wide variations globally and regionally (see Chap. 2)

Table 11–1 ESTIMATED RISKS FOR HIV TRANSMISSION FROM EXPOSURES TO INFECTED SOURCE CONTACTS

Exposure	Transmission Risk per 10,000 Exposures to HIV-Infected Sources
Blood transfusion	9,000
Shared needle for injection drug use	67
Receptive penile-anal intercourse	50
Nosocomial cutaneous needle injury	30
Receptive penile-vaginal intercourse	10
Insertive penile-anal intercourse	6.5
Insertive penile-vaginal intercourse	5
Receptive fellatio	1
Insertive fellatio	0.5
Cunnilingus	No documented transmission

Adapted from CDC (http://www.cdc.gov./mmwr/PDF/rr/rr5402.pdf).
Sexual transmission risks are for exposures without condom protection.

Transmission of HIV

Table 11–1 displays the estimated population-level risk of HIV transmission for single exposures to HIV-infected sources, ranging from 90% risk of exposure through blood transfusion to 0.005% (once for every 20,000 exposures) for the insertive partner in fellatio with an infected oral partner. Actual risks for individual exposures probably vary widely around these estimates.

- Sexual transmission accounts for most infections worldwide
  - Predominantly by penile-vaginal and penile-anal intercourse
  - Inefficient by oral-genital exposure; main risk is for oral-receptive partners in fellatio
  - Transmission by kissing occurs rarely, if ever
  - Transmission risk is strongly influenced by barrier protection, other STDs, male circumcision, HIV viral load, antiretroviral therapy, and other factors
- Parenteral transmission
  - Shared injection equipment among illicit drug users
  - Blood transfusion, organ donation; now rare worldwide
  - Nosocomial transmission, e.g., injury with contaminated instruments
- Mother-to-child (vertical) transmission
  - In utero (rare)
  - Perinatal during delivery
  - Postnatal, primarily through nursing
  - Now rare in industrialized countries and coming under control in many developing countries through maternal HIV screening, perinatal antiretroviral prophylaxis, and modified breastfeeding practices

Age

- In adolescents and adults, rates reflect ages for sexual risks and substance abuse
- Age distribution among 41,269 newly diagnosed HIV infections in the United States, 2008[*]

0 to 14 years	0.5%
15 to 19 years	4.5%
20 to 29 years	26.8%
30 to 39 years	25.5%
40 to 49 years	26.2%
≥50 years	16.5%

Sex

- Men and women accounted for 75% and 25%, respectively, of newly diagnosed HIV infections in the United States in 2008[*]
- Male and female rates are similar to each other in settings where heterosexual transmission dominates

Race and Ethnicity

- In 2008, 52% of newly diagnosed HIV infections in the United States* were in African Americans, who comprise 12% of the population
- Estimated annual incidence, 2006

	Rate per 100,000	Case ratio versus whites
White	11.5	
African American	83.7	7.3
Hispanic/Latino	29.3	2.5
Native American	14.6	1.3
Asian/Pacific Island	10.3	0.9

Sexual Orientation

- In the United States in 2008,[*] 57% of newly diagnosed HIV infections were in MSM, estimated to comprise 2–3% of the population
- Rare in women with exclusively female sex partners (in absence of other risks)

Injection Drug Use

- Injection drug users accounted for 13% of newly diagnosed HIV infections in the United States in 2008[*]

Heterosexual Exposure

- 32% of newly diagnosed HIV infections in the United States in 2008[*] were reported to result from heterosexual transmission

---

* At the time of publication, data on newly diagnosed HIV infections in the United States were available from 37 states with named reporting of HIV infections, regardless of stage. Named reporting of all HIV infections is now required in all 50 states and accurate nationwide data will become available as reporting patterns stabilize.

- True proportion of heterosexually transmitted cases probably is lower, because some infected persons deny potentially stigmatizing risk factors such as male homosexuality and injection drug use
- Heterosexually transmitted cases in the United States are heavily concentrated in racial and ethnic minorities and in eastern and southeastern urban areas

HISTORY AND CLINICAL MANIFESTATIONS

Epidemiologic History

- High-risk behavior or exposure to known HIV infection
- Demographic and other nonbehavioral markers
  - Residence in high-prevalence geographic area
  - Race or ethnicity other than white or Asian
  - Noninjection illicit drug use
  - Past or current bacterial STD or genital herpes
  - Commercial sex

Incubation Period

- Onset of primary HIV infection symptoms usually 10–20 days (range 7–28 days) after exposure
- Without antiretroviral therapy, AIDS (stage 3 HIV) typically develops 5–10 years after infection; rarely <1 year or >20 years

Clinical Classification of HIV Infection

CDC defines four clinical stages of HIV infection[†]

- Primary HIV infection
  - Positive blood test for HIV by PCR or other NAAT; *or* positive blood assay for HIV p24 antigen, *and*
  - HIV antibody negative
- Stage 1 HIV infection
  - CD4+ lymphocytes ≥500 cells/mm³ (or ≥29% of lymphocytes), *and*
  - No AIDS-defining condition (Table 11–2)

[†]Stage is determined by occurrence of an AIDS-defining condition, regardless of later resolution of the condition, or by the lowest documented CD4+ lymphocyte count. For example, a single CD4+ count of 480 cells/mm³ defines stage 2 in a patient with other CD4+ counts >500 cells/mm³; and following *Pneumocystis jiroveci* pneumonia, a patient has AIDS (stage 3) regardless of subsequent CD4+ lymphocyte counts.

- Stage 2 HIV infection
  - ○ CD4+ lymphocytes 200–499 cells/mm^3 (or 14–28% of lymphocytes), *and*
  - ○ No AIDS-defining condition (Table 11-2)
- Stage 3 HIV infection (AIDS)
  - ○ CD4+ lymphocytes <200 cells/mm^3 (or <14% of lymphocytes), *or*
  - ○ Occurrence of an AIDS-defining condition (Table 11–2)

Table 11–2 AIDS-DEFINING OPPORTUNISTIC DISEASES AND OTHER CONDITIONS IN HIV-INFECTED ADULTS

Respiratory candidiasis (bronchial, tracheal, pulmonary)
Esophageal candidiasis
Invasive cancer of the cervix
Extrapulmonary coccidioidomycosis
Extrapulmonary cryptococcosis
Intestinal cryptosporidiosis of >1 month duration
Cytomegalovirus (CMV) retinitis with vision loss, or CMV disease
  involving organs other than liver, spleen, or lymph nodes
HIV-related encephalopathy
Complicated herpes simplex virus infection
  - Chronic ulceration >1 month duration
  - Bronchitis
  - Pneumonia
  - Esophagitis
Extrapulmonary histoplasmosis
Intestinal isosporiasis of >1 month duration
Selected lymphomas
  - Burkitt lymphoma
  - Immunoblastic lymphoma
  - Primary brain lymphoma
Extrapulmonary nontuberculous mycobacterial infection (e.g.,
  Mycobacterium avium complex, *M. kansasii*)
Tuberculosis (*M. tuberculosis* or *M. bovis*)
*Pneumocystis jiroveci** pneumonia
Progressive multifocal leukoencephalopathy
Recurrent *Salmonella* septicemia
Cerebral toxoplasmosis
HIV-wasting syndrome

Adapted from Centers for Disease Control and Prevention, *MMWR* 2008;57(RR10). *Formerly *Pneumocystis carinii.*

Clinical Manifestations

Primary HIV Infection

- 50–80% of newly infected persons have symptomatic acute retroviral syndrome (ARS)[†]

- Primary clinical manifestations of ARS among symptomatic patients
    - Fever, typically 38–40°C (≥80% of patients; probably 90–100% if temperature is measured)
    - Sore throat/pharyngitis (40–70%)
    - Morbilliform rash (20–70%)
    - Malaise or fatigue (≥70%)
    - Generalized or cervical lymphadenopathy (35–70%)
    - Headache (30–60%)
    - Myalgias and/or arthralgias (40–70%)
    - Anorexia and/or weight loss (30–70%)
    - Gastrointestinal symptoms (nausea, vomiting, diarrhea) (20–50%)
    - Mucocutaneous ulcerations (primarily oral) (5–40%)

- Median duration of symptoms 10–14 days (range 7–42 days)

- Clinical picture is usually nonspecific, often resembling other common infections, especially infectious mononucleosis,[§] influenza, streptococcal pharyngitis, viral gastroenteritis, and others
    - About 70% of patients have all three among pharyngitis, fever, and rash
    - Even in patients at high risk with typical manifestations, other illnesses are more common than ARS

Stage 1-3 HIV/AIDS

- Following primary infection, most persons remain asymptomatic until opportunistic diseases supervene (Table 11–2)

- Common clinical manifestations with which patients may present in STD care settings include:
    - Persistent generalized lymphadenopathy
    - Constitutional symptoms (fever, weight loss, malaise)
    - Respiratory symptoms, e.g., cough, dyspnea
    - Chronic or persistent diarrhea
    - Seborrheic dermatitis (extensive or treatment-resistant)
    - Chronic herpetic ulcers (orofacial, genital, perianal)
    - Recurrent anogenital warts
    - Recurrent or treatment-resistant molluscum contagiosum, especially of face
    - Neuropsychological manifestations (e.g., peripheral neuropathy, dementia)
    - Skin lesions of Kaposi sarcoma

[†]Prospective studies suggest 75–80% of primary infections are symptomatic, but symptoms may be mild, and about 50% of retrospectively interviewed HIV seropositive patients recall ARS symptoms.
[§]In the early 1980s, many STD clinics and health care providers serving populations at risk for HIV anecdotally reported seeing many patients with heterophile-negative mononucleosis syndromes. In retrospect, many such persons had ARS.

- ○ Immune thrombocytopenia
- ○ Gingivitis
- ○ Candidiasis (oral, esophageal, or genital if recurrent or treatment-resistant)
- ○ Oral hairy leukoplakia
- ○ Oral aphthous ulcers
- ○ Fever of unknown origin

LABORATORY DIAGNOSIS

All STD clinical care facilities and providers in industrialized countries should have immediate access to assays for HIV antibody, preferably both laboratory-based enzyme immunoassay (EIA) and immediate point-of-care tests, plus a confirmatory antibody test such as Western blot. Tests should be available either directly or though consulting providers and laboratories for HIV p24 antigen (or an HIV antibody/p24 combination test), quantitation of CD4+ lymphocytes, and NAAT to detect HIV in blood, with determination of viral load. In resource-limited areas without immediate laboratory access, performance of two rapid point-of-care tests, by different manufacturers, is an accurate substitute for EIA with Western blot confirmation. The recently developed ("third generation") EIA and rapid test kits routinely employed in industrialized countries are ≥ 99% sensitive ≥3 months after infection (and approach 99% sensitivity by 6-8 weeks) for detection of antibody to HIV-1 subtype M, the dominant subtype worldwide and especially in industrialized countries. The p24 antigen/antibody combination test ("fourth generation") has ≥ 99% sensitivity ≥ 4 weeks after infection. Although some antibody tests, including Western blot, have reduced sensitivity (e.g., 80–90%) for detection of subtype O, other HIV-1 subtypes, and HIV-2, the prevalences of these HIV variants are low and sustained transmission is rare in the United States and most industrialized countries, so that test performance is not significantly affected at a population level. However, some patients with clinical syndromes or epidemiologic histories highly suggestive of HIV infection require additional testing for diagnosis, such as NAAT. Antibody and antigen assays for rare variants can be expected to reach the market soon.

HIV Antibody Tests

- Enzyme immunoassay
  - ○ Detects antibody to HIV nucleocapsid antigen p24 and envelope glycoproteins gp120 and gp41
  - ○ Numerous tests marketed by several manufacturers worldwide
  - ○ Antibody denotes infection with HIV, except passively acquired maternal antibody may be detected in newborns for up to 15 months
  - ○ Positive results require Western blot or other confirmatory test
  - ○ Seroconversion time: Recently developed ("third generation") tests detect both IgG and IgM antibody and become positive as soon as 10 days after infection, with estimated sensitivities ≥90% at 4 weeks and ≥95% at 6 weeks (perhaps ≥99%); sensitivity probably approaches 100% by 3 months
  - ○ Failure to seroconvert is observed rarely in patients with newly acquired HIV that progresses rapidly to overt AIDS; and in severe immune deficiencies characterized by impaired antibody production

- Rapid antibody tests
  - Detect antibody to same antigens as EIA, using whole blood (usually by finger stick), plasma, or oral crevicular fluid absorbed onto a pledget placed between cheek and gums
  - Point of care; results in 5–40 minutes
  - Several tests and manufacturers worldwide
  - Seroconversion time similar to third-generation EIA
  - Slightly reduced sensitivity and specificity (elevated rates of false-negative and false-positive results) versus EIA
  - Useful in settings in which immediate results are desirable, e.g., when follow-up is difficult (e.g., emergency and urgent care clinics, STD clinics)
  - Positive results on two rapid tests, by different manufacturers, have similar specificity for HIV diagnosis as EIA confirmed by Western blot; useful for field testing or if no EIA-capable laboratory is available (e.g., developing countries)
- Combination tests for HIV antibody and antigen ("fourth generation" HIV diagnostic tests)
  - Third-generation EIA combined with assay for p24 antigen
  - Several assays marketed worldwide, but as of this writing only one test was approved for use in the United States
  - Estimated sensitivity ≥99% ≥4 weeks after exposure
- Western blot
  - The primary confirmatory test, indicated for all positive EIA, EIA/p24, and single rapid test results
  - Indeterminate results are rare, due either to early seroconversion or, more frequently, nonspecific reactivity in atypical antibody bands, not indicating HIV infection

Virologic Tests

- HIV RNA/DNA NAAT
  - Detectable in plasma 7–10 days after acquisition; clinically useful in patients with suspected primary infection
  - Standard test to monitor plasma viral load, e.g., in following ARV drug therapy and to predict transmission risk and rate of progression of immunodeficiency
  - Pooled NAAT can efficiently detect early (pre-seroconversion) HIV infection when prevalence is sufficiently high for cost-effective testing
- HIV p24 antigen test
  - p24 antigen appears in blood 10–14 days after infection
  - Combined with third-generation EIA, shortens seroconversion window to ≤4 weeks

Lymphocyte Subset Analysis

- Quantitation of CD4+ (T4, "helper") lymphocyte count is primary determinant of immunodeficiency due to HIV infection; normal >600 cells per mm^3
- Determines stage of HIV infection, in combination with opportunistic AIDS-defining conditions (*See Clinical Classification of HIV Infection and Table 11-2*)

- Usually measured in tandem with NAAT to assess plasma viral load
  - CD4+ level is primary determinant of current state of immunodeficiency
  - Viral load predicts rate of progression of immunodeficiency

PREVENTIVE TREATMENT

Antiretroviral (ARV) drug therapy has potential roles in prevention of HIV infection in STD-related practices and settings. Other sources should be consulted for guidance on treatment of established HIV infection.

Postexposure Prophylaxis

Postexposure prophylaxis (PEP) with ARV drugs is effective in preventing HIV infection in animal models, and it appears to prevent infection in health care workers exposed in the workplace by traumatic or mucous membrane exposure to HIV-infected blood or secretions. Although no objective data have established efficacy in preventing infection by sexual or non-nosocomial blood exposure, PEP is frequently employed when patients present with histories of high-risk exposures. Based on animal models, effective PEP requires treatment within 72 hours of exposure, preferably within 24 hours. However, initiation later than 72 hours may be warranted in selected circumstances.

Criteria for Administration of Postexposure Prophylaxis

CDC and various investigators have published options for PEP in the United States, but the guidelines leave substantial leeway to define exposures with sufficient risk to warrant PEP. For example, commercial sex workers (CSWs) have widely varying HIV prevalences across geographic areas and population groups, allowing for divergent guidance for use of PEP following unprotected intercourse with CSWs. Similarly, there are wide geographic variations in the ability of risk markers such as race/ethnicity to predict the likelihood a partner is infected with HIV. In general, PEP is warranted if treatment can be initiated within 72 hours after unprotected vaginal or anal sex with a partner known to be infected or at substantial risk (e.g., MSM, injection drug user, some CSWs). Adaption of these general criteria to specific practices, clinics, and patients should consider:

- The nature of the sexual exposure, i.e., anal, vaginal, oral
- Successful use of condom or other barrier for vaginal or anal intercourse
- Known or likely infection status of the patient's partner, based on local epidemiology of HIV infection
- Treatment status and viral load of an HIV-infected source partner, if known
- Factors that affect transmission probability, e.g., circumcision, STDs, or sexual trauma
- Exposure of mucosal surfaces or non-intact skin to blood or genital or anorectal secretions (but not urine, saliva, sweat, or tears)
- Balance between HIV prevention potential and risk of serious ARV drug toxicity
- Availability and cost of selected ARV drugs
- Ability to test source partner of unknown status for HIV
- Local epidemiology of HIV resistance to available ARV drugs
- Patient desires and need for psychological support, e.g., following sexual assault

Drug Regimens for Postexposure Prophylaxis

CDC and other authorities list >15 regimens for which there is biologic plausibility for prevention. Treatment for 3–4 days can be initiated while confirming exposure, the HIV status of the source contact, and other factors that may influence a decision to complete a 4-week regimen. All decisions to administer PEP should be made in collaboration with an HIV prevention expert or using locally recommended ARV drug regimens, and continuing PEP generally should be supervised by an HIV prevention expert. Other sources should be consulted about side effects and other aspects of PEP.

At the time of publication, the following regimens** were readily available in the United States and commonly employed following high-risk sexual exposures. Different regimens often are used following community blood exposures or occupational exposures in health care workers.

- *Moderate-risk exposure,* e.g., unprotected vaginal intercourse with a partner at high risk for HIV but not known to be infected
  - Emtricitabine 200 mg/tenofovir 300 mg (Truvada) PO once daily for 28 days
- *High-risk exposure,* e.g., unprotected vaginal or anal intercourse with an infected or especially high-risk partner, such as an anonymous MSM
  - Efavirenz 600 mg/emtricitabine 200 mg/tenofovir 300 mg (Atripla) PO once daily for 28 days; *or*
  - Emtricitabine 200 mg/tenofovir 300 mg (Truvada) PO once daily *and* atazanavir (Reyataz) 300 mg once daily *and* ritonavir[††] (Norvir) 100 mg once daily for 28 days

Follow-up

- Antibody seroconversion and/or development of positive virological tests may be delayed if PEP is unsuccessful
  - Antibody testing periodically (e.g., every 2–4 weeks) until 6 months after exposure; plus (optionally) periodic NAAT or p24 antigen testing

Pre-exposure Prophylaxis

Recent years have seen considerable interest in pre-exposure prophylaxis (PrEP), with oral or vaginal ARV drug administration prior to risky sexual exposures, either intermittently or continuously. At the time of writing, one randomized, placebo-controlled trial had demonstrated substantial protection against HIV in sexually active women by tenofovir vaginal gel; several additional controlled trials were in progress.

PREVENTION

- Primary measure remains education and counseling to reduce high-risk behaviors
  - Maximum documented efficacy in HIV-infected persons

[**]The three regimens cited were recommended in 2010 by the Madison Clinic, Harborview Medical Center, Seattle, Washington, affiliated with the University of Washington. Madison Clinic is the primary HIV/AIDS treatment center in the Pacific Northwest region of the United States (http://depts.washington.edu/madclin/providers/index.html; accessed January 5, 2011).

[††]At recommended doses, ritonavir has little direct antiretroviral activity but enhances the activity of atazanavir and other protease inhibitors against HIV.

- ○ Efficacy of counseling has been difficult to document in uninfected individuals at risk
- ○ Vaccine research is underway but prospects for effective prophylactic immunization remain uncertain
- ○ Measures to limit nonintimate contact with HIV-infected persons (e.g., quarantine, restriction of employment) are ineffective and counterproductive

- Serological screening
  - ○ In the United States, all persons age 13–64 years should be tested at least once for HIV, regardless of risk, preferably with streamlined (opt-out) consent
  - ○ Benefits of screening include early diagnosis and referral for clinical care, as well as enhanced behavioral prevention efficacy when patients learn they are infected with HIV
  - ○ Among patients with STD or at risk, and in clinical settings where STDs are prevalent, most patients benefit from risk assessment and counseling, which are not precluded by routine opt-out testing
  - ○ Serological screening of donors is required to effectively prevent HIV transmission by blood products, organs, or artificial insemination
  - ○ Screening of pregnant women, combined with prophylactic ARV drug therapy, has markedly reduced frequency of neonatal HIV infection in industrialized countries

- Management of sex partners
  - ○ All infected patients should be advised to inform their needle-sharing and sex partners
  - ○ In the United States, local or state health department may assist in counseling and partner management

- Case reporting
  - ○ Named HIV case reporting, regardless of stage of infection, is now required by law in all states in the United States and in many countries
  - ○ Most health jurisdictions will assist in ensuring access of infected persons to clinical care and support services
  - ○ Case reporting assists in surveillance, prevalence monitoring, and design of prevention strategies

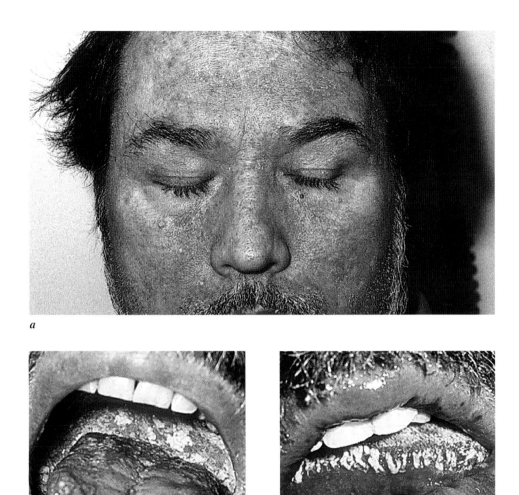

a

b   *c*

11–1. Clinical manifestations in a patient with AIDS. *a.* Facial seborrheic dermatitis; there is also a lesion of molluscum contagiosum below the right eye. *b.* Oral candidiasis of soft palate. *c.* Hairy leukoplakia of tongue.

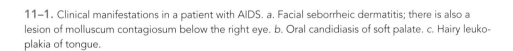

CASE

Patient Profile Age 33, gay male roofer

History Intermittent fever for 6 months, 15-lb weight loss; skin rash of face for 2 months; sore throat for 2 weeks; occasional unprotected sex with anonymous partners; repeatedly declined HIV testing over preceding decade ("I just didn't want to know")

Examination Erythematous facial rash with fine scale, involving forehead, nasolabial areas, and cheeks; umbilicated papular lesion below right eye; patchy white exudate on soft palate; hypertrophic striae of lateral aspects of tongue

Laboratory HIV antibody positive by EIA, confirmed by Western blot; VDRL negative; rectal tests for *N. gonorrhoeae* and *C. trachomatis* negative; hematocrit 34%, WBC 4,600 per mm^3 with reduced lymphocytes; CD4 lymphocyte count 122 per mm^3; plasma HIV-1 viral load 188,000 per mm^3; oral swab showed yeasts and pseudohyphae microscopically

Diagnosis HIV infection, stage 3 (AIDS) with oral candidiasis, oral hairy leukoplakia, seborrheic dermatitis, and facial molluscum contagiosum

Treatment ARV therapy initiated with indinavir, zidovudine, and didanosine; oral fluconazole; topical ketoconazole; molluscum contagiosum lesions treated with liquid nitrogen cryotherapy; trimethoprim/ sulfamethoxazole prophylaxis against *Pneumocystis jiroveci* pneumonia; pneumococcal and influenza immunizations

Comment After 4 months, the patient was asymptomatic, had regained his lost weight, and the seborrheic dermatitis and thrush had resolved. The CD4 lymphocyte count was 290 cells per mm^3 and the plasma HIV viral load was 5,000 per mm^3. Trimethoprim/suflamethoxazole was discontinued.

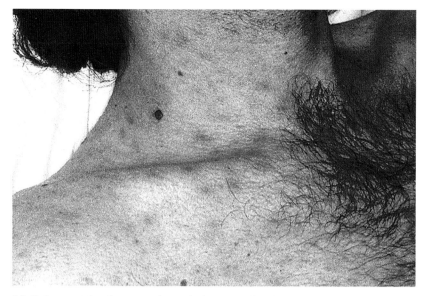

11–2. Primary HIV infection, with poorly demarcated erythematous macules and papules of the neck and upper trunk. (*Courtesy of David H. Spach, M.D. and Philip Kirby, M.D.*)

CASE

Patient Profile Age 24, unemployed gay man

History Sore throat, fever, and skin rash for 5 days; onset 10 days after unprotected receptive anal sex with unknown partner in a bath house

Examination Oral temperature 38.3°C; pharyngeal erythema, prominent tonsils with white exudate in crypts; cervical and axillary lymphadenopathy with 1–2 cm, slightly tender nodes; nonblanching maculopapular rash of upper trunk, neck, shoulders

Laboratory HIV antibody test negative; plasma p24 antigen and NAAT positive for HIV-1 RNA, 62,000 copies per mm³; hematocrit 36%, leukocyte count 7,600 per mm³ with 48% lymphocytes, platelet count 84,000 per mm³; CD4 lymphocyte count 322 per mm³; VDRL (negative); rectal NAAT for *N. gonorrhoeae* (positive) and *C. trachomatis* (negative); throat culture negative for *Streptococcus pyogenes* and *N. gonorrhoeae*

Diagnosis Primary HIV infection (CDC stage 1), subsequently stabilizing at stage 1; rectal gonorrhea

Treatment Patient declined antiretroviral therapy; ceftriaxone 250 mg IM, azithromycin 1.0 g PO

Comment Typical primary HIV infection syndrome, mimicking infectious mononucleosis with thrombocytopenia; HIV antibody test was positive 2 weeks later; fever, rash, and pharyngitis resolved over 2 weeks; clinical status stabilized to CDC stage 2 over 3 months: lymphadenopathy resolved, differential leukocyte count returned to normal, thrombocytopenia resolved, CD4 lymphocyte count was 665 per mm³, and plasma HIV-1 viral load 5,500 copies per mm³

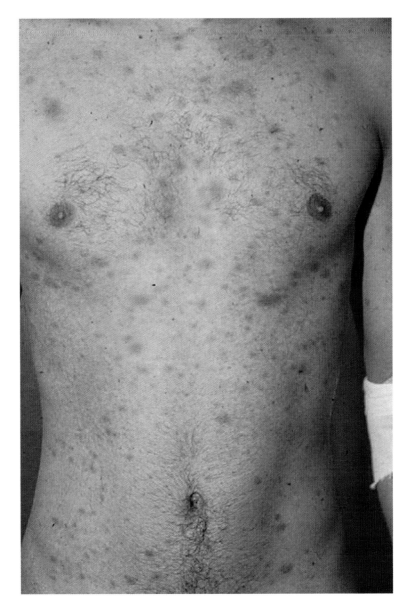

11–3. Generalized maculopapular rash in primary HIV infection. (*Courtesy of Armin Rieger, MD.*)

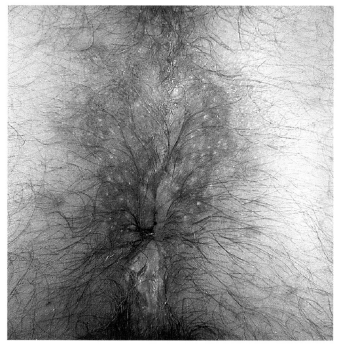

a

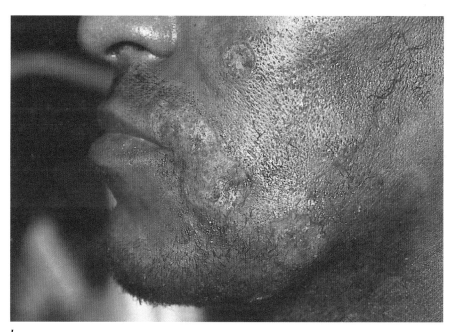

b

11–4. Chronic herpes due to HSV-2 in HIV-infected patients. *a.* Extensive perianal ulceration due to HSV-2; such lesions can be very debilitating due to pain. (*Courtesy of Steven J. Medwell, M.D.*) *b.* Chronic facial ulcers, atypically due to HSV-1. (*Courtesy of Philip Kirby, M.D.*) Such lesions usually respond to treatment with valacyclovir, famciclovir, or acyclovir. If present >1 month, such lesions define overt AIDS (CDC stage 3). (Also see Fig. 8-18.)

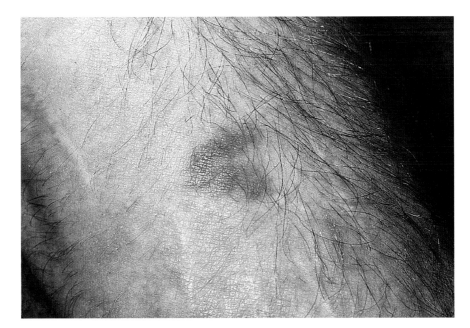

11–5. Macular Kaposi sarcoma lesion of the forearm in a patient with AIDS. Kaposi sarcoma lesions usually are nodular (see Fig. 11–6), with violaceous or brown color due to vascular proliferation and hemosiderin deposition, but the appearance is highly variable. Kaposi sarcoma is caused by human herpesvirus type 8 (HHV-8) (see Chap. 12). (*Courtesy of Philip Kirby, M.D.*)

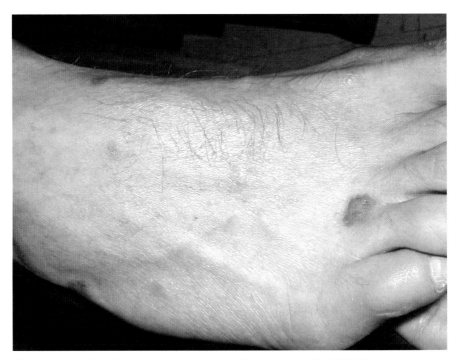

11–6. Nodular Kaposi sarcoma skin lesions of the foot in a man with AIDS. Similar lesions were widely distributed, especially on the trunk, and were the first recognized manifestation of the patient's HIV infection. The lesions regressed with ART. (*Courtesy of Robert Harrington, M.D.*)

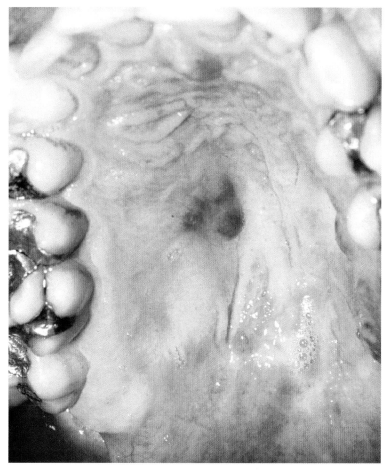

11–7. Kaposi sarcoma of the palate in AIDS. Kaposi sarcoma often presents with oral lesions. (*Courtesy of James P. Harnisch, M.D.*)

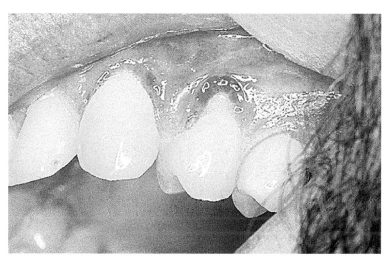

11–8. Gingivitis in AIDS. Gum retraction and gingivitis are common oral findings in HIV infection.

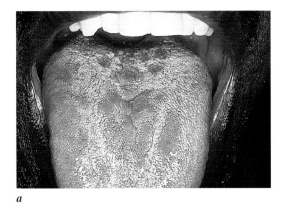

a

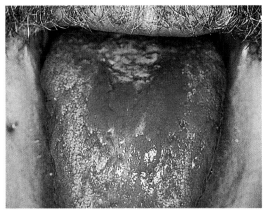

b

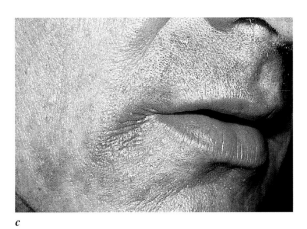

c

11–9. Oral candidiasis in AIDS; not all cases present with white patchy exudate typical of thrush (see Fig. 11–1b). *a.* Erythematous candidiasis of tongue. *b.* Erythematous and pseudomembranous candidiasis of tongue. *c.* Angular cheilitis due to *Candida albicans*. (*Courtesy of David H. Spach, M.D.*)

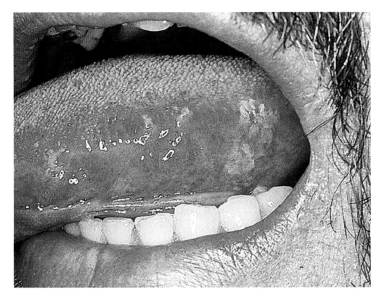

11–10. Hairy leukoplakia of the tongue in HIV infection; early lesions mimic premalignant leukoplakia and may lack the prominent linear pattern seen in advanced cases (compare with Fig. 11–1c). Hairy leukoplakia is a manifestation of Epstein-Barr virus infection and often responds to therapy with high-dose valacyclovir or famciclovir.

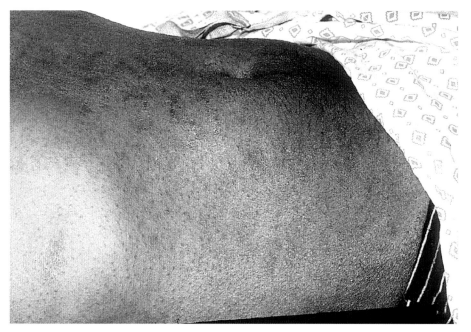

11–11. AIDS-related ichthyosis. HIV-infected persons with advanced immunodeficiency often complain of dry skin and generalized pruritus, with evidence of dyshidrosis. Advanced cases present with overt ichthyosis, with dry, raspy skin, fine scale, and hyperpigmentation. (*Courtesy of Philip Kirby, M.D.*)

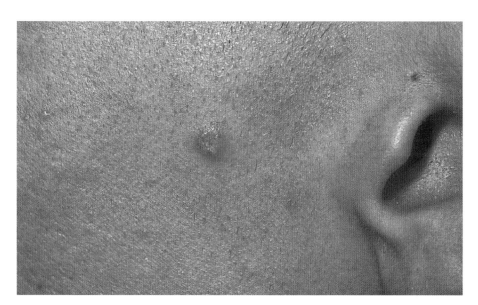

11–12. Molluscum contagiosum of the cheek in a patient with AIDS. Facial molluscum or warts may result from recrudescence of latent infection, perhaps dating to childhood, due to cellular immunodeficiency (Also see Fig. 11-1a). (*Courtesy of Philip Kirby, M.D.*)

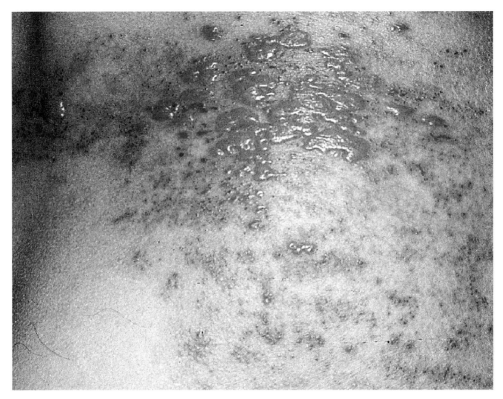

11–13. Herpes zoster (shingles) in a patient with CDC stage 2 HIV infection (CD4+ lymphocyte count 320 cells per mm^3). (*Courtesy of David H. Spach, M.D.*)

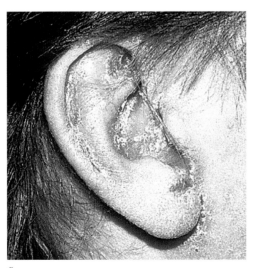

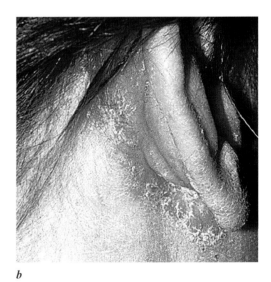

a   *b*

11–14. Advanced seborrheic dermatitis in a patient with AIDS. Seborrheic dermatitis occasionally is sufficiently severe to suggest herpes zoster. This case resolved promptly with topical ketoconazole therapy. (*Courtesy of David H. Spach, M.D.*)

SUGGESTED READING

Centers for Disease Control and Prevention. HIV/AIDS home page. http://www.cdc.gov/hiv/. Accessed January 5, 2011. *Extensive information about HIV/AIDS in the United States, including CDC's annual surveillance report, clinical practice and prevention guidelines, and links to international HIV/AIDS resources.*

Centers for Disease Control and Prevention. Recommendations for postexposure interventions to prevent infection with hepatitis B virus, hepatitis C virus, or human immunodeficiency virus, and tetanus in persons wounded during bombings and other mass-casualty events—United States, 2008. *MMWR Recomm Rep.* 2008;57(RR-6):1-19. http://www.cdc.gov/mmwr/preview/mmwrhtml/rr5706a1.htm?s_cid =rr5706a1_e . Accessed January 5, 2011. *Guidance from CDC on regimens and strategies available for PEP as of 2008.*

Centers for Disease Control and Prevention. Revised recommendations for HIV testing of adults, adolescents, and pregnant women in health-care settings. *MMWR Recomm Rep.* 2006;55(RR-14):1-17. http://www.cdc.gov/mmwr/preview/mmwrhtml/rr5514a1.htm. Accessed January 5, 2011. *Recommendations for routine screening for HIV in the United States.*

Chu C, Selwyn PA. Diagnosis and initial management of acute HIV infection. *Am Fam Physician.* 2010; 15:1239-44. *A succinct review of the clinical manifestations and management of ARS.*

Glynn JR, et al. Herpes simplex virus type 2: a key role in HIV incidence. *AIDS.* 2009;31:1595-8. *An editorial and succinct review; an excellent introduction to the importance of HSV-2 and other STDs in HIV transmission.*

Karim SSA, et al. Global epidemiology of HIV-AIDS. *Infect Dis Clin N Am.* 2007;21:1-17. *A comprehensive review of the topic; the introductory paper in an issue devoted to the state of the art and science of HIV/AIDS.*

Moses S. Male circumcision: a new approach to reducing HIV transmission. *CMAJ.* 181;E134-5. http://www.cmaj.ca/cgi/reprint/181/8/E134. Accessed January 5, 2011. *A summary succinct review of the data documenting the efficacy of male circumcision in Africa to prevent HIV, by one of the leading researchers in the field.*

Volberding PA, Deeks SG. Antiretroviral therapy and management of HIV infection. *Lancet.* 2010;376: 49-62. *A review by leading authorities of drug options, controversies on criteria for initiating ARV therapy, and HIV/AIDS management.*

12

Blood-Borne Viruses: Viral Hepatitis, Epstein-Barr Virus, Cytomegalovirus, and Others

Hepatitis B virus (HBV) is a blood-borne virus that also is shed in genital secretions and transmitted by sexual contact and vertically to infants born to infected mothers, as well as by exposure to blood through transfusion and shared ejection equipment. In industrialized countries, sexually transmitted HBV infection is especially common among men who have sex with men (MSM). Most HBV infections resolve spontaneously, but chronic persistent infection can lead to chronic hepatitis and cirrhosis with hepatic failure, and predisposes to hepatocellular carcinoma.

Hepatitis C virus (HCV) is transmitted almost exclusively by exposure to infected blood. The importance of sexual transmission has been controversial, but it is now understood that sexual transmission contributes little to overall incidence and prevalence. There is no direct evidence of transmission by semen or other genital secretions, and most heterosexual partners of HCV-infected persons remain uninfected unless they also have overt blood exposure, e.g., through shared injection equipment. However, sexual transmission has been clearly documented in MSM who participate in traumatic anorectal sexual practices, especially if they are also infected with HIV. Few HCV infections cause overt acute hepatitis, but most infections persist chronically and often progress to cirrhosis and hepatic failure.

Hepatitis A virus (HAV) can be transmitted by sexual practices that foster oral exposure to feces, but not by blood exposure. In adults, infection typically causes acute, symptomatic hepatitis. Chronic infection does not occur, so that sustained sexual transmission is limited by the brief time of infectivity during acute hepatitis.

Epstein-Barr virus (EBV), the agent of infectious mononucleosis, causes chronic, persistent infection and is secreted in saliva and genital secretions. Historically infectious mononucleosis was characterized as a "kissing disease," reflecting the potential of transmission by saliva. However, it is now understood that most cases in sexually active young adults are acquired through sexual intercourse, and acute EBV infection should be considered an STD. Accordingly, sexual history and screening tests for other STDs should be routine in the management of teens and young adults with mononucleosis.

Cytomegalovirus (CMV) in adults is acquired largely through sexual exposure or from infected children who shed the virus in saliva. Most infections are asymptomatic but some result in heterophile-negative mononucleosis or other syndromes. Other blood-borne viruses with variable frequencies of sexual transmission in different populations and settings include human herpesvirus type 8 (HHV-8), hepatitis D virus (HDV), and human T-cell lymphotropic virus types 1 and 2 (HTLV-1 and -2). All of these cause chronic infections that usually remain asymptomatic but can be transmitted, often sexually, for prolonged periods and perhaps for life. Several types of adenovirus occasionally are sexually transmitted, often by orogenital practices, and can cause nongonococcal urethritis (NGU). All enteric viruses can be transmitted by sexual practices that foster fecal-oral exposure.

HEPATITIS A

Epidemiology and Transmission

- Estimated annual U.S. incidence 25,000 cases in 2007, primarily through nonsexual transmission
- Declining rates in the past 2 decades, with rising rates of routine immunization in childhood
- 29–33% of the U.S. population has serological evidence of past infection
- Endemic in many developing countries, primarily spread through fecal-oral contamination, either by personal contact or environmental contamination
- Sexually transmissible by practices that foster oral exposure to feces; the dominant transmission mode among MSM
- Fecal shedding and transmission are limited to acute infection (2–6 weeks)

Clinical Manifestations

- Incubation period 3–5 weeks
- Most adults have nausea, malaise, jaundice; 90% of infections in children are asymptomatic
- Main signs are tender hepatomegaly and jaundice, but anicteric cases are common
- Clinical resolution occurs and hepatic enzymes usually decline to normal within 6 weeks (rarely up to 3 months) after onset
- Rare cases of fulminant hepatitis with liver failure
- No chronic infection (in contrast to hepatitis B and C)

Diagnosis

- Often suspected by typical clinical presentation and exposure history
- Elevated hepatic enzymes (e.g., alanine aminotransferase) and bilirubin
- Serology for anti-HAV antibody
  - IgM anti-HAV detectable 3–5 weeks after acquisition; diagnostic of acute infection
  - IgG anti-HAV detectable within 6–10 weeks and persists indefinitely

Treatment

- Supportive care
- No generally available antiviral therapy is known to be effective

Prevention

- Immunization with anti-HAV vaccine (two doses separated by 6–12 months) is indicated for susceptible (seronegative) MSM, and for all persons anticipating high-risk exposure (e.g., travel to high-incidence environments), or exposure to known case
- Passive immunization with immune globulin 0.02 mL/kg body weight IM (simultaneous with first vaccine dose) is recommended for patients who present within 2 weeks of known exposure
- Avoiding practices that foster oral-fecal exposure (e.g., analingus) helps prevent sexual transmission

HEPATITIS B

Epidemiology and Transmission

- Estimated annual U.S. incidence 43,000 new infections in 2007
- Declining in the past 2 decades due to rising immunization rates
- 4.3–5.6% of U.S. residents have been infected
- Prevalence of chronically infected persons in the United States estimated at 800,000–1,400,000 persons
- Endemic at high rates in most developing countries, depending on extent of immunization
- Transmitted by blood exposure, sexual contact, and perinatally
- Sexual transmission probably is most efficient by anal intercourse, less so by vaginal intercourse, probably rare by orogenital exposure
- In the United States and most high-income countries, rates are highest in MSM and injection drug users (IDU)

Clinical Manifestations

- Incubation period 6–12 weeks
- Acute infection often (35–70%) symptomatic
- Main symptoms are nonspecific (e.g., fever, malaise, anorexia, nausea) without clinically obvious hepatitis
- Occasionally jaundice, tender hepatomegaly
- Serum sickness-like prodrome, with skin rash, polyarthritis, or manifestations of cryoglobulinemia occur in 15–20% of cases
- Chronic infection usually asymptomatic, with or without biochemical or biopsy evidence of chronic active hepatitis
- Cirrhosis and hepatocellular carcinoma are late complications

Diagnosis

- Primarily based on serological tests for HBV surface antigen (HBsAg), antibody to surface antigen (anti-HBs), and antibody to core antigen (anti-HBc)
  - ◦ HBsAg indicates acute infection or chronic active hepatitis and potential infectivity
  - ◦ Anti-HBs and anti-HBc usually indicate resolved or inactive infection
  - ◦ Anti-HBs, in absence of anti-HBc, suggests prior immunization
- Hepatitis B e antigen (HBeAg) denotes enhanced infectivity and high probability of transmission

Treatment

- Acute infection: symptomatic therapy only
- Chronic infection: natural and recombinant interferons, ribavirin, and other antiviral drugs
- Manage in consultation with hepatologist or other expert

Prevention

- Immunization with HBsAg-based vaccine is cornerstone of prevention; recommended routinely in childhood with catch-up vaccination of adults at risk
  - ◦ Adult vaccine dose: 20 mg IM at 0, 1, and 6 months; however, any schedule that achieves 3 doses ≥1 month apart within 1–2 years appears to be effective
  - ◦ Vaccinate all MSM, IDU, teens, adults with STD, and health care workers who were not immunized in childhood
  - ◦ In populations at highest risk (e.g., MSM, IDU) it is cost-effective to simultaneously screen with serology and administer first vaccine dose; vaccination is safe if previously infected or immunized; initial vaccine dose may be given simultaneously with serological test
- High-risk exposure to known HBV infection: start immunization with HBV vaccine and simultaneously administer HBV immune globulin 0.06 mL/kg IM (usually 3–5 mL); repeat HBV immune globulin in 1 month if vaccination not given or if compliance with vaccine schedule is in doubt
- Condoms are effective in preventing transmission by vaginal or anal intercourse

HEPATITIS C

Epidemiology and Transmission

- Estimated annual U.S. incidence 17,000 infections in 2007 (50% decline since 2000)
- 1.3–1.9% of U.S. residents have been infected
- Estimated 12,000 deaths annually in the United States due to HCV-related chronic liver disease; HCV-related hepatic failure is the most common indication for liver transplantation
- Most cases acquired by blood exposure
- Sexual transmission is infrequent and inefficient except by exposures characterized by substantial blood exposure
- Despite common perceptions of HCV infection as an STD, sexual transmission is well documented only among MSM who participate in traumatic anorectal sex (e.g., "fisting"), perhaps especially if HIV-infected

Clinical Manifestations

- Most acute infections are subclinical
- Occasional overt hepatitis
- Chronic persistent hepatitis occurs in two-thirds of persons with HCV infection; usually asymptomatic until onset of cirrhosis or hepatic failure

Diagnosis

- EIA for anti-HCV antibody, confirmed by anti-HCV recombinant immunoblot assay
- HCV RNA, detected by reverse-transcriptase PCR or branch-chain DNA, confirms active infection
- Liver function tests and biopsy to guide clinical management

Treatment

- Acute infection: symptomatic support
- Chronic infection: natural and recombinant interferons, ribavirin
- Clinical response depends in part on HCV subtype
- Manage in consultation with hepatologist or other expert

Prevention

- Anti-HCV screening of blood donors
- Avoidance of blood exposure, e.g., control of injection drug use, no shared injection equipment
- Counsel MSM to avoid traumatic rectal sexual practices
- Condoms and sex partner selection probably have little impact on transmission
- Routine serological screening of IDU and persons exposed to unscreened blood products
- Testing not recommended for sex partners of infected persons in absence of blood exposure risk

EPSTEIN-BARR VIRUS

Epidemiology and Transmission

- Ubiquitous; 90–95% of adults are seropositive
- Most frequently transmitted in childhood; 50% seropositive by age 5
- At least 90% of seropositive persons shed virus intermittently in saliva, oropharynx, genital secretions
- In teens and adults, acquisition is primarily by sexual intercourse; primarily through saliva in childhood
- Genital shedding of EBV increased in presence of inflammatory STDs (e.g., gonorrhea)

Clinical Manifestations

- Usually subclinical, especially in children
- Clinically evident infectious mononucleosis occurs in up to 50% of teens or adults with primary infection

- Symptomatic mononucleosis: fever, pharyngitis, generalized lymphadenopathy, malaise; typical duration 2–8 weeks
- Long-term complications include non-Hodgkin lymphoma, nasopharyngeal carcinoma, and other malignancies; rarely Guillain-Barre syndrome, immunopathologic disorder, cerebellar dysfunction, and numerous others
- Opportunistic disease in AIDS and other immunodeficiency disorders, including oral hairy leuko-plakia, non-Hodgkin lymphoma, and other malignancies

Diagnosis

- Positive assay for "heterophile" antibody (e.g., Monospot)
- EBV-specific antibodies:
  - IgG and IgM antibody to EBV viral capsid antigen (VCA)
  - IgG antibody to EBV nuclear antigen
- Virologic detection of EBV in blood by PCR; useful in diagnosis of atypical infections and management of EBV-related malignancies
- Routine blood count may reveal atypical lymphocytosis

Treatment

- EBV is inhibited by acyclovir and related drugs, but little clinical benefit has been demonstrated except in selected settings (e.g., treatment of hairy leukoplakia in AIDS)
- Infectious mononucleosis: symptomatic therapy only; corticosteroids may speed improvement in severe cases
- Oral hairy leukoplakia in patients with AIDS: acyclovir or valacyclovir

Prevention

- Condoms may be protective, but no data available

CYTOMEGALOVIRUS

Epidemiology and Transmission

- In the United States, CMV seroprevalence 10–15% in teens, increasing to about 50% by age 35, with substantial geographic and demographic variation; higher prevalences in developing countries
- Transmitted by exposure to genital secretions, saliva, blood
- Vertical (maternal–neonatal) transmission
- Superinfection with new strains is common
- Nonsexual transmission from infected children to adult caregivers, especially in crowded settings (e.g., nursery, daycare, preschool)

Clinical Manifestations

- >95% of CMV infections in adults are asymptomatic
- Occasional mononucleosis-like syndrome or granulomatous hepatitis
- Congenital transmission usually is subclinical

- Overt congenital disease may be most frequent following primary maternal infection during pregnancy; can cause severe multisystem disease with neurodevelopmental disability or subtle manifestations (e.g., neurosensory hearing loss)
- Severe, often life-threatening manifestations of CMV are common in persons with profound immunodeficiency (e.g., AIDS, organ transplantation), inluding retinitis, pneumonia, esophagitis, colitis, encephalitis, and others

Diagnosis

- Virological identification of CMV by culture, PCR, or antigen detection in blood, urine, or infected tissues
  - CMV is often identified in chronic, nonpathological infection; quantitative virus levels may be useful to establish clinical significance
- Serology is of limited utility due to high prevalence of chronic subclinical infection
- Characteristic histopathology on biopsy or cytology

Treatment

- Acute infection: Symptomatic management
- Symptomatic congenital infection: Ganciclovir (e.g., 6 mg/kg IV every 12 hours for 6 weeks) may be helpful
- Opportunistic infection in immunodeficient patients: Ganciclovir, valganciclovir, foscarnet, cidofovir, or CMV-immune globulin have documented or potential benefit
- Manage in consultation with an expert

Prevention

- Condoms may help prevent sexual transmission
- Vaccine research promising, but no vaccine currently available
- Preventing primary CMV infection in pregnant women (e.g., condoms, no new partnerships, avoidance of occupational exposure to young children) may reduce risk of in utero transmission and congenital infection

OTHER VIRUSES

Human Herpesvirus Type 8

HHV-8 is the cause of Kaposi sarcoma, both in persons with AIDS and in endemic Kaposi sarcoma typically diagnosed in older persons without HIV infection. HHV-8 has been identified in saliva and semen, and epidemiologic studies suggest the virus frequently is sexually transmitted, especially in MSM. However, the epidemiology has not been completely characterized and other modes of transmission may occur. Primary infection can cause manifestations similar to those of infectious mononucleosis and acute HIV infection, but most infections probably are asymptomatic.

Hepatitis D Virus

HDV is an "incomplete" virus that replicates only in the presence of HBV, resulting in clinical exacerbations of hepatitis B. HDV is transmitted primarily by blood contact; sexual transmission may occur but apparently is infrequent.

Human T-Cell Lymphotrophic Viruses

Human T-cell lymphotropic virus type 1 (HTLV-1) causes adult T-cell leukemia/lymphoma and tropical spastic paraparesis and myelopathy. HTLV-2 is not clearly associated with known pathology. HTLV-1 and HTLV-2 have epidemiologic parallels with HBV and HCV; blood exposure and sexual contact probably explain most cases.

Adenovirus

Adenovirus type 19 and several other types are primarily upper respiratory viruses, but can cause acute conjunctivitis with urethritis and sometimes are sexually transmitted, probably by orogenital contact. Adenovirus is responsible for 2–3% of cases of NGU.

Enteroviruses

Enteroviruses and other enteric viruses are often transmitted by sexual practices that foster oral exposure to feces.

SUGGESTED READING

Casper C. New approaches to the treatment of human herpesvirus 8–associated disease. *Rev Med Virol.* 2008;5:321-9. *A comprehensive review of the epidemiology and treatment of HHV-8 and its association with Kaposi sarcoma.*

Coonrod D, et al. Association between cytomegalovirus seroconversion and upper genital tract infection among women attending a sexually transmitted diseases clinic: a prospective study. *J Infect Dis.* 1998;177:1188-93. *A careful analysis documenting 10–12% annual incidence of primary CMV infection in seronegative women attending an STD clinic, and association with acquisition of other STDs.*

Crawford DH, et al. A cohort study among university students: identification of risk factors for Epstein-Barr virus seroconversion and infectious mononucleosis. *Clin Infect Dis.* 2006;43:276-82. *Documentation of sexual transmission of acute EBV infection, one of two papers by the same investigators; also see* J Infect Dis. *2007;195:474-82.*

Hakki M, Geballe A. Cytomegalovirus. Chapter 25 in KK Holmes, et al., eds. *Sexually Transmitted Diseases.* 4th ed. New York, NY: McGraw-Hill; 2008:439-51. *Review of CMV pathology, clinical manifestations, epidemiology, and transmission.*

Lemon SM, et al. Viral hepatitis. Chapter 29 in KK Holmes, et al., eds. *Sexually Transmitted Diseases.* 4th ed. New York, NY: McGraw-Hill; 2008:509-43. *Review of HAV, HBV, and HCV from the perspective of sexual transmission.*

Staras SA, et al. Influence of sexual activity on cytomegalovirus seroprevalence in the United States. *Sex Transm Dis.* 2008;35:472-9. *Documentation of the association of CMV seropositivity with sexual behavior in a nationally representative sample, supporting the important role of sexual transmission.*

Cutaneous Infestations

13

Pediculosis Pubis

Infestation with the crab louse (*Phthirus pubis*), or pediculosis pubis, is usually acquired through sexual contact with an infested person, but some cases probably result from exposure to shared clothes or bedding. *P. pubis* is adapted to survival in the pubic region, and *Pediculus humanus* to the head and body, by extremities adapted to grasping pubic hair or head and body hairs, respectively. Pruritus is common, but many patients are asymptomatic until eggs (nits) or lice are noticed. Maculae ceruleae, localized discoloration due to intracutaneous bleeding at sites of attachment, are rare but pathognomonic. Complications of pediculosis pubis are virtually unknown, and infestation is more a nuisance than a significant threat to health. Infestation is a marker of STD risk, and patients should be screened for other STDs.

EPIDEMIOLOGY

Incidence and Prevalence

- Very common, but no reliable statistics available
- Diagnosed in 2–5% of patients attending some STD clinics

Transmission

- Transmission occurs primarily by pubic area apposition with an infested person
- *P. pubis* is slowly motile and survives <24 hours without a blood meal, limiting nonsexual transmission; however, occasional cases may be transmitted through contaminated bedding or clothing

Age

- No predilection; reflects sexual behavioral risks

Sex

- No special predilection

HISTORY

Incubation Period

- Ova (nits) hatch in 5–10 days
- Hatched lice mature in 6–9 days and begin laying nits
- Symptoms may be delayed by several days or weeks, as pruritus is partly a consequence of allergy

Symptoms

- Visible nits or lice often are the only complaint
- Pubic area itching
- Lice appear nonmotile and may seem to adhere to skin, sometimes mistaken for scabs

Epidemiologic History

- Behavioral and population risks for STD
- Sexual contact with known case
- Sometimes communal living, typically in settings of poor hygiene

PHYSICAL EXAMINATION

- Nits, attached at base of hair, are the most common sign of infestation
- Lice may be difficult to identify, particularly in dark-skinned patients
- Infestation usually limited to the pubic area, but sometime extends to thighs or trunk
- Eyelashes and eyebrows are occasionally involved, scalp rarely if ever
- Maculae ceruleae are pathognomonic but uncommon

LABORATORY DIAGNOSIS

- If diagnosis in doubt on visual inspection, suspected nits and lice may be examined microscopically

DIAGNOSTIC CRITERIA

- Identification of nits or lice

TREATMENT

Regimens of Choice

- Permethrin 1% cream rinse
- Pyrethrins with piperonyl butoxide
- Either treatment is applied to pubic area, intergluteal folds, and all skin surfaces from knees to waist, and to any other visibly infested areas except eyelashes
- Eyelash infestation: apply occlusive ophthalmic ointment to eyelid margins *bid* for 10 days

Alternative Regimens

- Resistance of pubic, body, and head lice to insecticides is widespread and increasing; use alternative if infestation persists after initial treatment
  - Malathion 0.5% lotion applied for 8–12 hours then rinsed
  - Ivermectin 250 μg per kg body weight PO, repeated in 2 weeks (limited clinical experience)

PREVENTION

- Main prevention strategies are sex partner selection and maintenance of personal hygiene
- Sex partners should be routinely treated

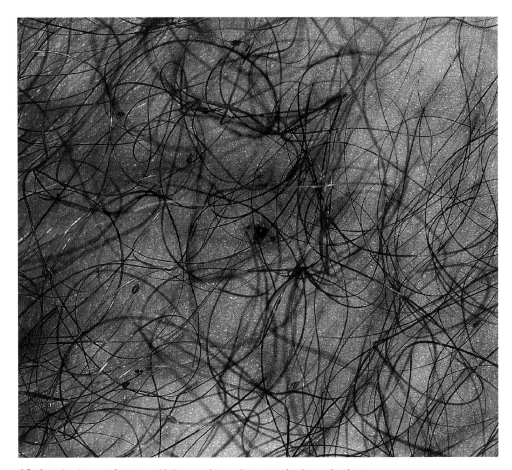

13–1. Pubic louse infestation; *Phthirus pubis* and nits attached to pubic hairs.

CASE

Patient Profile Age 33, male construction worker

History Pubic area itching for 1 week; noticed "white spots" clinging to pubic hair 1 day earlier; occasional causal sexual contacts

Examination Nits and typical crab lice in pubic hair; otherwise normal

Laboratory Urine NAAT for *Chlamydia trachomatis* and *Neisseria gonorrhoeae*, serological tests for syphilis and HIV (all negative)

Diagnosis Pediculosis pubis

Treatment Permethrin 1% cream rinse

Partner Management Advised to inform partners and recommend attendance for clinical evaluation, or self-treatment with over-the-counter preparations, e.g., pyrethrins with piperonyl butoxide lotion

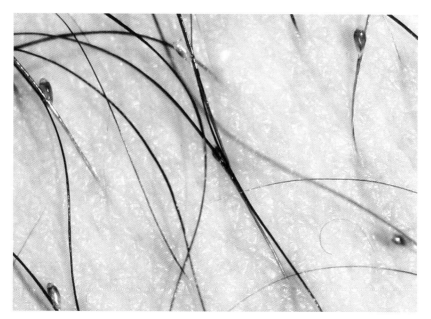

13–2. *Phthirus pubis* nits (eggs) attached to pubic hairs. (*Cho SB, Kim HS: Images in clinical medicine. Pediculosis of the pubis, NEJM. Feb 19;360(8):e11, 2009. With permission.*)

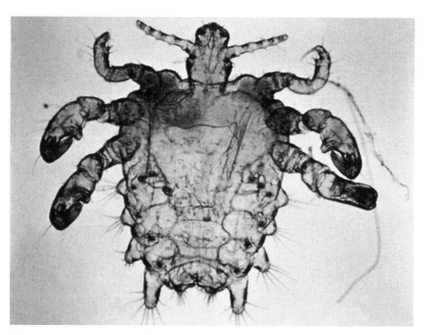

13–3. *Phthirus pubis*, the pubic louse, also called the crab louse. (*Reproduced with permission from the World Health Organization [WHO]*).

SUGGESTED READING

Leone PA. Pubic lice and scabies. Chapter 46 in KK Holmes, et al., eds. *Sexually Transmitted Diseases.* 4th ed. New York, NY: McGraw-Hill; 2008:839-51. *A comprehensive review in the definitive textbook on STDs.*

Leone PA. Scabies and pediculosis pubis: an update of treatment regimens and general review. *Clin Infect Dis.* 2007;44(Suppl 3):S153-9. *Review of the data in support of CDC's 2006 STD treatment guidelines.*

14

Scabies

Scabies is cutaneous infestation with the itch mite, *Sarcoptes scabiei*. The organism is highly infectious and transmitted by close personal contact. Sexual exposure is a frequent mode of transmission, but infestation also is commonly acquired through shared bedding and clothing and sometimes nosocomially, especially in skilled nursing facilities and other chronic care settings. Scabies is among the most common dermatoses observed in persons attending STD clinics. The primary clinical manifestation is an intensely pruritic papular eruption, often with secondary excoriations; hyperkeratotic, nodular, vesicular, or bullous lesions sometimes occur. Most clinical manifestations result from hypersensitivity to the mite and its feces and ova, so that symptoms typically develop 2–4 weeks after acquisition of the first infestation but often within 1–2 days in subsequent infestations. In addition, hypersensitivity may result in persisting symptoms for a few weeks following successful scabicidal treatment. Secondary staphylococcal or streptococcal infection is common. An infrequent but important complication is crusted ("Norwegian") scabies, characterized by extensive hyperkeratosis and large numbers of mites, sometimes seen in AIDS patients or persons taking high doses of corticosteroids.

EPIDEMIOLOGY

Incidence and Prevalence

- No accurate incidence data
- Epidemics tend to recur in 10–30 years cycles
- Diagnosed in up to 5% of STD clinic patients

Transmission

- Skin-to-skin contact or exposure to infested fomites, e.g., bed linens or shared clothing
- Sexual exposure may be the most common mode of acquisition in young adults
- Nonsexual contact accounts for many cases in households and other settings (e.g., hospitals, nursing homes, shelters)

Age

- All ages affected

Sex

- No special predilection

Sexual Orientation

- No special predilection

Other Risk Factors

- Settings of poor hygiene and crowding, e.g., homeless shelters
- Nosocomial transmission to health care workers sometimes occurs, especially if initial case has especially high organism load, as in crusted scabies

HISTORY

Incubation Period

- Typically 2–4 weeks from infestation to first symptoms for first episode
- Often as brief as 1–2 days for subsequent infestations, due to hypersensitivity

Symptoms

- Localized or generalized skin rash with intense itching, often worse at night or exacerbated by bathing
- Pruritus sometimes occurs on apparently uninvolved skin surfaces
- Absence of itching is evidence against scabies

Epidemiologic History

- Behavioral risks for STD
- History of exposure to scabies
- Communal living, especially in settings of poor hygiene

PHYSICAL EXAMINATION

- Papular skin rash, usually with secondary excoriations
- Most commonly involved sites are flexor surfaces of elbows, axillae, hands, finger webs, waist, ankles, dorsal surfaces of feet, genitals, buttocks, inguinal and gluteal folds
- Genital lesions often seen in patients seeking care in STD clinics
- Often 0.5–1.0-cm linear lesions that mark the paths of burrowing mites, sometimes with a leading black dot or small vesicle that marks the mite's location
- Occasional vesicular, nodular, scaling, bullous lesions or eczematous plaques
- Secondarily infected pustules or localized cellulitis are common
- Crusted (Norwegian) scabies manifested by marked hyperkeratosis, fissures, and secondary infection

LABORATORY DIAGNOSIS

- Microscopy of scrapings of lesions, obtained with a scalpel blade and mixed with 10% KOH solution or mineral oil, showing mites, ova, or scybala (fecal pellets)
- Microscopy is insensitive; multiple scrapings often are necessary for diagnosis
- Biopsy occasionally required

DIAGNOSTIC CRITERIA

- Diagnosis usually is suspected on the basis of symptoms and clinical appearance
- Application of water-based ink followed by wiping with alcohol may highlight mites' intracutaneous burrows ("burrow ink test")
- Microscopic confirmation is recommended, especially for atypical cases
- Assessment of response to treatment (therapeutic trial) sometimes is helpful, but clinical response may be slow

TREATMENT

Regimens of Choice

- Permethrin 5% cream, applied to entire skin surface from neck down, washed off after 8–14 hours
- Ivermectin 250 μg per kg body weight PO, repeated in 2 weeks; regimen of choice for crusted scabies
- Symptomatic improvement may be delayed ≥2 weeks after successful scabicidal treatment, due to hypersensitivity to slowly resorbed mites, ova, and scybala

Alternative Regimen

- Lindane 1% lotion (1 oz) or cream (30 g) applied to entire skin surface below the neck, washed off after 8 hours; because of risk of toxicity, should be used only if regimens of choice are unavailable or ineffective

Ancillary Measures

- Launder or dry-clean bed linens and all clothing used within 48 hours prior to treatment
- Antihistamines (e.g., diphenhydramine, hydrazine) or other antipruritus drugs may speed symptomatic relief
- Antibiotics may be indicated if secondary bacterial infection is present

PREVENTION

- Mainstays are avoidance of high-risk sexual exposures, shared living quarters in settings of poor hygiene, and direct personal contact with infested persons
- Routinely treat sex partners and persons sharing living quarters with infested persons

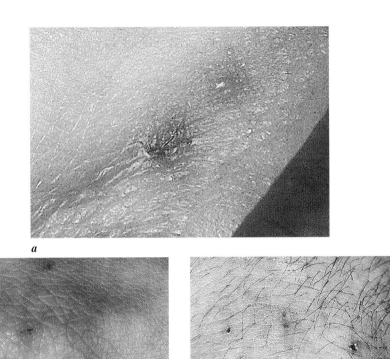

a

b

c

14–1. Scabies. *a.* Papules of finger web; one lesion has been excoriated. *b.* Papules of knuckle; note dark line across papule, which yielded diagnostic scrapings. *c.* Excoriations on extensor surface of elbow.

CASE

Patient Profile Age 19, male carpenter

History Intense "itching all over" for 2 weeks, worse at night; onset 4 weeks after intercourse with an unknown female partner

Examination Erythematous papules and excoriations of hands, elbows, around waist; genital examination normal

Differential Diagnosis Scabies, eczema, dermatitis herpetiformis, contact dermatitis

Laboratory Microscopic examination of lesion scrapings demonstrated ova and feces of *S. scabiei*; screening urine NAAT) for *Chlamydia trachomatis* and *Neisseria gonorrhoeae*, VDRL, HIV serology; positive for *C. trachomatis*

Diagnosis Scabies; urethral chlamydia (asymptomatic)

Treatment Permethrin 5% cream; counseled to launder bed linens and clothing used in preceding 48 hours; azithromycin 1.0 g PO, single dose

Comment Symptoms and rash subsided gradually over 10 days; incidental chlamydial infection illustrates importance of scabies as STD risk

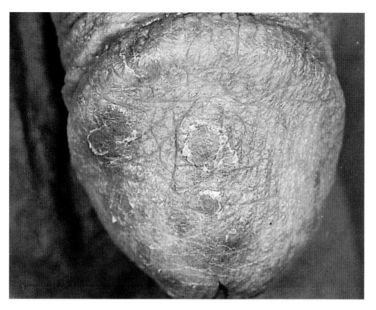

14–2. Scabies of glans penis. Note similarity to secondary syphilis (see Fig. 5–14). psoriasis (see Figs. 22–5 and 22–6), and keratoderma blennorrhagica of reactive arthritis (see Figs. 17-2 and 17-3).

CASE

Patient Profile Age 37, homeless man living in a communal shelter

History Pruritic rash for 2 weeks, worse at night; no recent sexual exposure; scabies or itching reported to be common among other shelter residents

Examination Exfoliating papules on glans and shaft of penis; numerous papules, nodules, excoriations of trunk and extremities

Differential Diagnosis Scabies, secondary syphilis, keratoderma blennorrhagica (reactive arthritis), psoriasis

Laboratory Scrapings negative for scabies; VDRL, HIV serology, urine NAAT for *N. gonorrhoeae* and *C. trachomatis* (all negative)

Diagnosis Scabies

Treatment Permethrin 5% cream

Comment The penis is a common site of scabies lesions, perhaps especially among infested persons who seek care in STD clinical settings. Despite negative scrapings, the diagnosis of scabies was secure based on clinical presentation and epidemiologic history. The patient's symptoms and rash resolved over 2 weeks; the therapeutic response helped confirm diagnosis. The local health department inspected the shelter, diagnosed five additional cases of scabies, and arranged for treatment of all residents and simultaneous laundry of all clothing and bed linens.

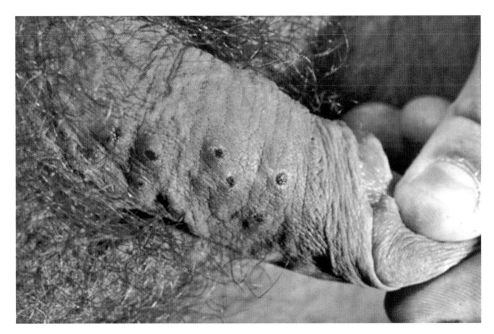

14–3. Scabies mimicking genital herpes. The patients presented with painful, pruritic lesions of the penis, which he had excoriated by scratching. Herpes was suspected but diagnostic tests were negative, and scabies was diagnosed by microscopy of scrapings of similar lesions on the elbows and hands. (*Courtesy of Michael L. Remington.*)

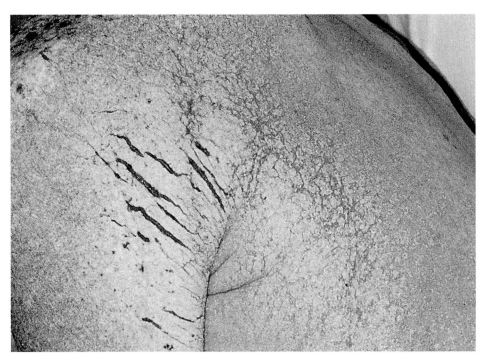

14–4. Crusted (Norwegian) scabies in a man with AIDS. (*Courtesy of David H. Spach, M.D.; reprinted with permission from Spach DH, Fritsche TR. Norwegian scabies in a patient with AIDS. New Engl J Med. 1994;331:777.*)

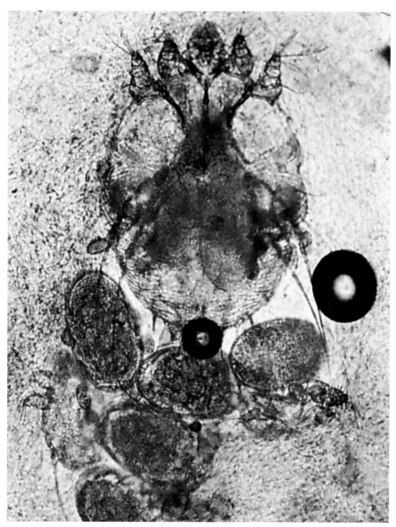

14–5. *S. scabiei* with ova, scraped from a scabies skin lesion. (*Reproduced with permission from KK Holmes, et al, eds. Sexually Transmitted Diseases. 3rd ed. New York, NY: McGraw-Hill; 1999.*)

SUGGESTED READING

Currie BA, McCarthy JS. Permethrin and ivermectin for scabies. *N Engl J Med.* 2010;362:717-25. *Review of the current primary treatment options for scabies.*

Leone PA. Pubic lice and scabies. Chapter 46 in KK Holmes, et al., eds. *Sexually Transmitted Diseases.* 4th ed. New York, NY: McGraw-Hill; 2008:839-51. *A comprehensive review in the definitive textbook on STDs.*

• Section Five

Clinical Syndromes

15

Nongonococcal Urethritis

By definition, nongonococcal urethritis (NGU) is urethritis not caused by *Neisseria gonorrhoeae*; it is the most common diagnosis among men presenting to STD clinics. The term nonspecific urethritis (NSU) is synonymous with NGU and is used preferentially in some countries. Postgonococcal urethritis is NGU following successful treatment of gonorrhea, with an etiologic spectrum similar to that of *de novo* NGU, and occurs in about 25% of men with gonorrhea treated with cephalosporins without azithromycin or a tetracycline.

Chlamydia trachomatis causes 25–35% of cases of initial, nonrecurrent NGU, and about 10–20% of cases are caused by the recently characterized *Mycoplasma genitalium*. *Ureaplasma urealyticum* may cause 10–30% of cases, but conflicting data exist. It is only recently that *U. urealyticum* has been differentiated from the ubiquitous, apparently nonpathogenic *U. parvum*, and forthcoming research that distinguishes these two organisms may help elucidate the role of *U. urealyticum* in NGU and other genital disorders. Neither *C. trachomatis*, *M. genitalium*, nor *U. urealyticum* can be identified in half or more of affected men. *Trichomonas vaginalis*, herpes simplex virus, usually type 1 (HSV-1), and certain strains of adenovirus each account for 2–5% of cases in recent series. Men with NGU with signs that suggest herpes, such as typical cutaneous lesions, prominent erythema and edema of the meatus, or severe dysuria, should be treated with drugs for HSV as well as the usual bacterial etiologies. When urethritis persists or recurs after initial therapy, repeat treatment should include coverage for *T. vaginalis*. Some men with NGU without an identifiable pathogen give histories of insertive fellatio, without other recent sexual exposures, suggesting that oropharyngeal flora may cause some cases. It is unknown (and unstudied) whether normal or unidentified organisms in partners' vaginal or rectal flora may explain some cases of NGU. *Escherichia coli* or other fecal bacteria occasionally cause NGU following insertive anal intercourse. The differential diagnosis of urethritis also includes urethral foreign bodies and periurethral fistulas, but both are rare. Anecdotal reports suggest that NGU is commonly misdiagnosed as a nonsexually acquired urinary tract infection (UTI) by clinicians unfamiliar with the clinical syndrome. However, UTI is rare in men under 40 years old.

The main complications of NGU are those caused or triggered by *C. trachomatis*, including acute epididymitis and reactive arthritis, but epididymitis has not been linked to nonchlamydial NGU. There is no evidence that urethral stricture results from NGU; most such cases in the pre-antibiotic era probably were due to gonorrhea or traumatic therapies such as irrigation with caustic compounds like silver nitrate or potassium permanganate. Although *C. trachomatis* carries obvious health implications for men's female sex partners, NGU without identified pathogens has not been associated with morbidity in either the female or male partners of affected men. The female partners of men with nonrecurrent NGU should be routinely treated, primarily to cover *C. trachomatis* and *M. genitalium*, but the need for treatment is uncertain if these have been excluded and *T. vaginalis* is absent. It is unknown whether treatment benefits the receptive partners in oral or anal sex, but it is commonly provided.

Persistent or recurrent NGU is a common and often vexing problem for patients and providers alike. Repeated relapses are frequent in some men, often without sexual reexposure, and *C. trachomatis* or other recognized pathogens are rarely identified. Recurrent NGU occasionally may be associated with nonbacterial prostatitis or chronic pelvic pain syndrome, but usually the prostate is not involved. There is no evidence that alcohol, highly spiced foods, changes in sexual frequency, or Valsalva maneuver ("strain") can cause acute or recurrent urethritis, notwithstanding past beliefs to the contrary. A common error in management of men with persistent or recurrent symptoms is failure to document urethral inflammation by examination for urethral leukocytes. Without objective evidence of urethral inflammation, symptoms alone usually are not indications for repeated antibiotic therapy. Even when urethritis is documented, it is possible that some persistent or recurrent cases result from noninfectious immunologic mechanisms. Much about NGU and its related syndromes remains to be explained by future research. For example, there is renewed interest in the relationship between STDs and later prostate gland morbidity because of recent studies showing transient elevations of prostate-specific antigen in some men with gonorrhea or chlamydial urethritis, although not in men with nonchlamydial NGU.

EPIDEMIOLOGY

Incidence and Prevalence

- Accurate data unavailable
- Accounts for 10–30% of new problem visits by men to STD clinics

Transmission

- Initial episodes of NGU usually are acquired sexually, but exceptions may occur
- Oral-genital exposure probably accounts for some cases of nonchlamydial NGU
- Recurrent or persistent NGU probably results primarily from relapse, but reinfection often cannot be excluded

Age

- Most cases age 15–35 years
- All ages susceptible

Sex and Sexual Orientation

- By definition, NGU occurs only in men
- Mucopurulent cervicitis may be female counterpart in some instances (see Chap. 18)
- In MSM, *C. trachomatis* accounts for <10% of cases, and many cases are associated with oral-genital exposure

HISTORY

Incubation Period

- Typically 1–3 weeks

Symptoms

- Urethral discharge is the primary symptom
- Dysuria usually is mild, often absent; sometimes described as urethral itching or tingling
- Severe dysuria suggests viral etiology (HSV, adenovirus)
- Urinary urgency, frequency, or pelvic or perineal pain are uncommon; they suggest cystitis, chronic pelvic pain syndrome, or prostatitis

Epidemiologic History

- Usually new sex partner, but exceptions are common
- Some cases occur in monogamous men, perhaps caused by partners' normal vaginal, rectal, or oral flora

PHYSICAL EXAMINATION

- Urethral discharge
  - Typically mucoid or mucopurulent; occasionally purulent
  - Variable in amount, from spontaneous to scant amounts expressed by urethral compression; may be apparent only after several hours without urination
  - Some patients lack demonstrable discharge
- Scant clear mucus sometimes is observed normally in men without urethritis, especially after sexual arousal or prolonged interval since urination
- Occasional meatal erythema or edema ("meatitis"), especially in cases associated with HSV or adenovirus
- HSV urethritis may be associated with localized tenderness along penile shaft at sites of intra-urethral herpetic lesions
- Penile venereal edema (painless edema of penis, without erythema) sometimes accompanies urethritis or genital herpes

DIAGNOSIS

Documentation of Urethritis

- Clear history of abnormal urethral discharge; *or* observation of abnormal discharge (see History and Physical Examination)

and

- Evidence of inflammatory response in the urethra:
  - Gram-stained smear of external urethral exudate or endourethral swab, showing elevated PMNs

or

  - Positive leukocyte esterase test on initial 30 mL of voided urine

Microbiologic Tests

- Tests for *C. trachomatis* and *N. gonorrhoeae*, preferably by NAAT (see Chaps. 3 and 4)
- Testing for *M. genitalium* by NAAT not yet routinely recommended nor widely available, but may become useful
- Testing for *T. vaginalis* by NAAT not yet routinely recommended nor widely available, but may become useful
- Tests for *U. urealyticum* are not recommended
- Urine culture for uropathogens may be useful in selected settings, e.g., for NGU following insertive anal intercourse or if urgency or urinary frequency are present
- Test for HSV (NAAT or culture) if clinical findings or exposure suggest herpes

Recurrent or Persistent NGU

After symptomatic resolution, urethritis recurs within 6 weeks in 10–20% of men following chlamydial NGU and in 20–30% after nonchlamydial NGU.

- Confirm urethral inflammation by Gram-stained smear showing PMNs *or* positive leukocyte esterase test
- Microbiologic evaluation
  - Repeat NAATs for *C. trachomatis* and *N. gonorrhoeae* rarely are productive unless patient reexposed to untreated partner
  - NAAT for *T. vaginalis* may be useful if available
  - Urine culture for uropathogens may be useful
  - Tests for *M. genitalium* or *U. urealyticum* are not readily available in most settings but may be useful in some patients

TREATMENT

Initial NGU*
Treatments of Choice

- Azithromycin 1.0 g PO, single dose
- Doxycycline 100 mg PO *bid* for 7 days

Alternative Regimens

- Erythromycin base 500 mg PO *qid* (or equivalent alternate erythromycin formulation) for 7 days
- Ofloxacin 300 mg PO *bid* for 7 days
- Levofloxacin 500 mg PO once daily for 7 days

---

*Nonrecurrent NGU, i.e. no previous episode in past 3 months.

Suspected HSV Urethritis

A viral etiology of NGU, often due to HSV or adenovirus, is suggested by presence of mucocutaneous lesions consistent with genital herpes, or by severe dysuria, prominent erythema or edema of the meatus, or conjunctivitis.

- Acyclovir, valacyclovir, or famciclovir (see Chap. 8) in addition to azithromycin or doxycycline

Persistent or Recurrent NGU

- First recurrent or persistent episode[†]
  - If initial episode treated with azithromycin, use doxycycline as above
  - If doxycycline used initially, use azithromycin

  plus
  - Metronidazole 2.0 g PO, single dose, or tinidazole 2.0 g PO, single dose
- Subsequent recurrent episodes[†]
  - For second and subsequent recurrences, some experts recommend moxifloxacin 400 mg PO once daily for 7 days.[‡]
  - More prolonged courses (2–6 weeks) of fluoroquinolone antibiotics (e.g., ofloxacin, levofloxacin, ciprofloxacin) have been employed by some clinicians, especially when NGU may be accompanied by prostatitis; no controlled studies are available
  - Persistent or recurrent symptoms of urethritis should not be treated with antimicrobial drugs unless urethritis is confirmed by urethral leukocytosis
  - Consider evaluation for prostatitis and chronic pelvic pain syndrome

PREVENTION

- As for chlamydial infection and gonorrhea (see Chaps. 3 and 4)
- Examine and treat female sex partners of patients with nonrecurrent NGU for presumptive chlamydial infection
- The standard practice is to treat partners of men with initial nonchlamydial NGU, but benefits to prevent either reinfection of the index case or morbidity in partners are unknown
- Repeated treatment generally is not recommended for partners of men with recurrent NGU
- Recommend condoms for new or casual sexual encounters

[†]Within 3 months of prior episode.
[‡]Moxifloxacin is consistently active against *Mycoplasma genitalium*, which may explain some cases of persistent NGU after treatment with doxycycline or azithromycin.

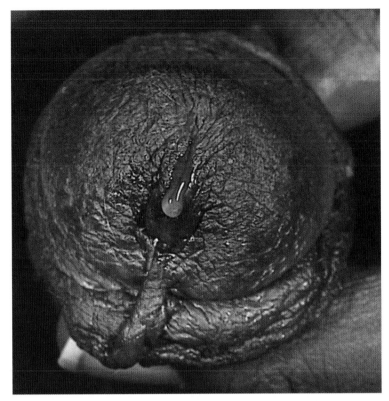

15–1. Mucopurulent urethral discharge in NGU.

CASE

Patient Profile Age 26, graduate student and teaching assistant, heterosexual

History Urethral "itching" and intermittent urethral discharge for 7 days; began a new sexual relationship 6 weeks earlier

Examination Mucopurulent urethral discharge

Differential Diagnosis Urethritis; probable NGU, rule out gonorrhea

Laboratory Urethral Gram stain showed 15–20 PMNs per 1000× field and scant mixed bacterial flora, without GND; urethral NAATs for *C. trachomatis* and *N. gonorrhoeae* (both negative); VDRL and HIV serology negative

Diagnosis Nonchlamydial NGU

Treatment Azithromycin 1.0 g PO, single dose

Other The patient was counseled about the sexually acquired nature of his infection and the need to arrange for examination and treatment of his partner. Expedited partner therapy (EPT) is a consideration for partner management when partners are not likely to attend in person, but has been rigorously studied only for confirmed gonorrhea, chlamydial infection, and trichomoniasis.

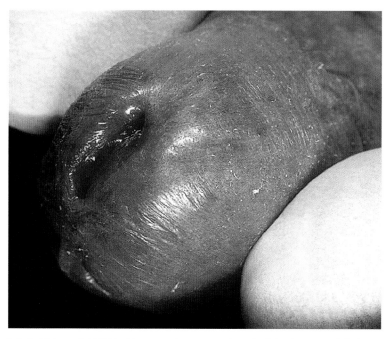

15–2. Chlamydial NGU with scant, clear, mucoid urethral discharge, and slight meatal erythema.

CASE

Patient Profile Age 34, flight attendant, MSM

History Urethral discharge for 5 days; no dysuria or other symptoms; regularly had unprotected insertive anal and oral sex with his steady partner; occasional sex with other men, usually but not invariably with condoms; denied receptive anal intercourse in preceding year; negative HIV test 4 months earlier

Examination Scant, clear, mucoid urethral discharge; slight meatal erythema

Differential Diagnosis Urethritis: probable NGU, rule out gonorrhea; possible coliform urethritis

Laboratory Urethral Gram stain showed 10–12 PMNs per 1000× field, without GND; urethral NAATs for *N. gonorrhoeae* (negative) and *C. trachomatis* (positive); pharyngeal culture for *N. gonorrhoeae* (negative); urine culture for UTI pathogens (negative); VDRL and HIV serology (both negative)

Diagnosis Chlamydial NGU

Treatment Doxycycline 100 mg PO *bid* for 7 days

Comment Scant clear appearing urethral moisture was found on examination. Doxycycline was prescribed, rather than azithromycin, to cover both *C. trachomatis* and some potential causes of coliform urethritis while awaiting urine culture result. Advised to refer partner for evaluation; EPT has not been validated in MSM, in whom high risk for other STDs supports personal examination.

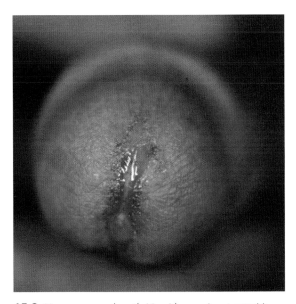

15-3. Nongonococcal urethritis with prominent meatitis. Tests for *C. trachomatis* and *N. gonorrhoeae* were negative. Meatitis, characterized by prominent dysuria and meatal erythema, raises the probability of viral etiology, such as HSV or adenovirus. There were no cutaneous lesions and urethral culture for HSV was negative.

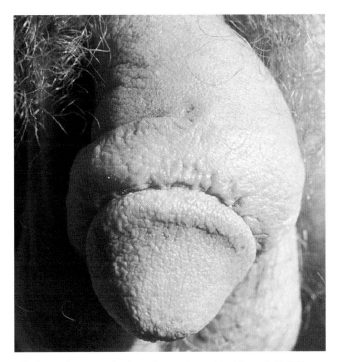

15–4. Penile venereal edema in a patient with chlamydial NGU. (Compare with Figs. 4–8, 8–4a, and 8–6.)

SUGGESTED READING

Bradshaw C, et al. Etiologies of nongonococcal urethritis: bacteria, viruses, and the association with orogenital exposure. *J Infect Dis.* 2006;193:336-45. *The results of a large observational study documenting current etiologies based on NAAT for several common and uncommon bacteria and viruses.*

Gaydos C, et al. *Mycoplasma genitalium* compared to chlamydia, gonorrhoea and trichomoniasis as an aetiological agent of urethritis in men attending STD clinics. *Sex Transm Infect.* 2009;85:438-40. *An observational study in an inner-city STD clinic, demonstrating* M. genitalium *as the likely etiology in about 30% of men with NGUs.*

Krieger JN. Prostatitis syndromes: causes, differential diagnosis, and clinical management. Chapter 61 in KK Holmes, et al., eds. *Sexually Transmitted Disease.* 4th ed. New York, NY: McGraw-Hill; 2008:1147-74. *A comprehensive review with discussion of the differentiation of prostatitis from urethritis. It also addresses chronic pelvic pain syndrome, often a manifestation of genitally focused anxiety in men fearful about STD.*

Martin DH. Urethritis in males. Chapter 59 in KK Holmes, et al., eds. *Sexually Transmitted Diseases.* 4th ed. New York, NY: McGraw-Hill; 2008:1107-26. *An authoritative review of urethritis, with emphasis on clinical management.*

Schwebke JR, et al. Re-evaluating the treatment of nongonococcal urethritis: emphasizing emerging pathogens—a randomized clinical trial. *Clin Infect Dis.* 2011;52:163-70. *A multicenter trial with results suggesting that doxycycline may be superior to azithromycin against* C. trachomatis, *and that azithromycin is modestly effective against* M. genitalium.

Yokoi S, et al. The role of *Mycoplasma genitalium* and *Ureaplasma urealyticum* biovar 2 in postgonococcal urethritis. *Clin Infect Dis.* 2007;45:866-71. *The first study of the etiology of postgonococcal urethritis using nucleic acid amplification for diagnosis, documenting roles for* C. trachomatis, M. genitalium, *and* U. urealyticum. *An accompanying editorial (Manhart LE, et al.* Clin Infect Dis. *2007;45:872-4) provides useful perspective.*

Epididymitis

Acute epididymitis results from ascending lower genital tract infection, analogous to the pathogenesis of pelvic inflammatory disease in women. *Chlamydia trachomatis* and *Neisseria gonorrhoeae* cause most cases in men under 35 years old. Coliform bacteria or other traditional uropathogens are common causes in men older than 35 years, the insertive partners in anal intercourse, and in men with anatomic anomalies or recent urethral instrumentation. Tuberculosis and fungal infections such as coccidioidomycosis or cryptococcosis are occasionally implicated; tuberculosis in particular should be considered in patients with or at risk of HIV. Noninfective epididymitis can be caused by vasculitis and, rarely, certain drugs such as the anti-arrhythmic drug amiodarone. All teens and young adults with acute testicular pain should be evaluated for testicular torsion, a surgical emergency. Epididymitis is usually unilateral and rarely explains vague or bilateral testicular pain without tenderness, induration, or swelling; men with such complaints often have chronic pelvic pain syndrome or prostatitis.

EPIDEMIOLOGY

Incidence and Prevalence

- Medical claims data suggest that 0.3–0.5% of males age 14-35 are diagnosed with epididymitis per year
- No accurate statistics available; epididymitis probably complicates ≤1% of urethral gonococcal and chlamydial infections
- In heterosexual men <35 years old, 50–70% due to *C. trachomatis* and 5–40% due to *N. gonorrhoeae*, depending on local incidences of chlamydial infection and gonorrhea
- In men >35 years old, most cases are due to coliforms or *Pseudomonas* and are associated with bacterial UTI

Transmission

- As for *C. trachomatis* and *N. gonorrhoeae*
- Coliform urethritis and epididymitis can be sexually acquired by anal intercourse

Age

- Most sexually acquired cases age 15–35 years

Sexual Orientation

- Men who participate in insertive anal intercourse may be at elevated risk

Other Risk Factors

- Urinary tract instrumentation
- Anatomic abnormalities of lower urinary tract
- Bacterial prostatitis
- Tuberculosis in HIV-infected persons
- Amiodarone therapy
- Contrary to past beliefs, valsalva maneuver ("strain") with reflux of urine into epididymis does not cause epididymitis

HISTORY

Incubation Period

- Not well studied; onset often follows urethral chlamydial, gonococcal, or coliform infection by several days to a few weeks

Symptoms

- Testicular pain and swelling, usually unilateral, ranging in severity from mild to severe
- Sometimes inguinal pain
- Symptoms usually develop over 1–2 days, but onset may be perceived as sudden
- Fever may occur but is uncommon
- Urethritis reflects underlying etiology, i.e., usually mild or absent in chlamydial infection, prominent in gonorrhea
- Urinary urgency or frequency, without discharge, suggest bacterial UTI
- Bilateral testicular pain, without urethritis, UTI, tenderness, or other examination findings are rarely due to epididymitis; consider chronic pelvic pain syndrome or prostatitis

Epidemiologic History

- Often high-risk sexual exposure, as for chlamydia or gonorrhea (see Chaps. 3 and 4)

PHYSICAL EXAMINATION

- Symptoms and examination abnormalities usually are unilateral
- Epididymal and testicular enlargement

- Tenderness, often severe, often localized to epididymis but may involve entire testicle as well as epididymis (epididymo-orchitis)
- Scrotal erythema in severe cases
- Signs of urethritis often present, e.g., purulent or mucopurulent urethral discharge (see Chaps. 3, 4, and 15)

LABORATORY TESTS

Evaluation for Lower Genital Tract Infection

- Evaluate as described for NGU, chlamydial infection, and gonorrhea (see Chaps. 3, 4, and 15)
- In coliform epididymitis, midstream urine may show pyuria by microscopy or leukocyte esterase test

Microbiologic Tests

- NAATs for *C. trachomatis* and *N. gonorrhoeae* (see Chaps. 3 and 4)
- Urine culture for uropathogens

Other Tests

- Immediate assessment of blood flow (e.g., Doppler study or radionuclide scan) in patients at risk for testicular torsion:
  - Age ≤25 years, especially teens
  - Sudden onset
  - Absence of urethritis or pyuria
  - Testicle elevated in scrotal sac
- Blood culture if febrile

DIAGNOSIS

- Epididymal or testicular tenderness and swelling plus evidence of urethritis or bacterial urinary tract infection establishes the diagnosis with high reliability
- Differential diagnosis includes the "four Ts"
  - Torsion: Common in teens, many of whom also are at risk for STD
  - Tumor, i.e. testicular cancer
  - Trauma, sometimes without history of injury
  - Tuberculosis
- Other uncommon causes include cryptococcosis and other systemic fungal infections, vasculitis syndromes, amiodarone toxicity

TREATMENT

Suspected Sexually Acquired Epididymitis

- Ceftriaxone 250 mg IM plus doxycycline,[*] 100 mg PO *bid* for 10 days

Nonsexually Acquired Infective Epididymitis

- Ofloxacin[†] 300 mg PO *bid* for 10 days
- Levofloxacin[†] 500 mg PO once daily for 10 days

PARTNER MANAGEMENT AND PREVENTION

- As for chlamydial infection and gonorrhea (see Chaps. 3 and 4)

---

[*] Prior to microbiologic diagnosis, doxycycline is preferred over azithromycin in order to enhance coverage for coliform infection.

[†] Ofloxacin or levofloxacin is preferred over ciprofloxacin and other fluoroquinolones in order to cover *Chlamydia trachomatis* prior to microbiologic diagnosis.

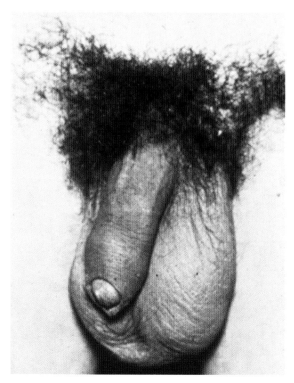

16–1. Acute epididymitis of right testicle; mucopurulent urethral discharge is present. (*Courtesy of Walter E. Stamm, M.D.*)

CASE

Patient Profile Age 28, married electrical engineer

History Mild left testicular pain for 2 days, becoming severe with swelling for 6 hours; denied urethral discharge and dysuria; sexual exposure 1 month earlier with new female partner

Examination Scrotum warm, skin erythematous; testicle indurated, enlarged to twice normal size; marked tenderness, maximal posteriorly, extending into spermatic cord; mucopurulent (white) urethral discharge

Differential Diagnosis Acute epididymitis; possible trauma, torsion, cancer, tuberculosis, or other granulomatous inflammation

Laboratory Gram-stained urethral smear showed >15 PMNs per 1000× (oil immersion) microscopic field, without GND; leukocyte esterase test on midstream urine (negative); urethral cultures sent for *C. trachomatis* (positive) and *N. gonorrhoeae* (negative); midstream urine culture (no growth)

Diagnosis Chlamydial epididymitis

Treatment Ceftriaxone 250 mg IM (single dose) plus doxycycline 100 mg PO *bid* for 10 days

Partner Management Advised to refer wife and his new partner for treatment for presumptive chlamydia infection

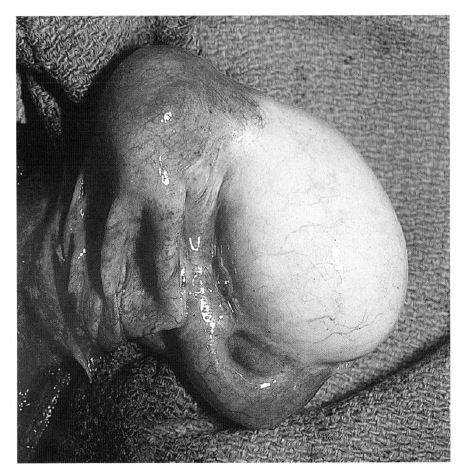

16–2. Acute epididymitis due to amiodarone; the epididymis is enlarged and erythematous; surgery was performed because tumor was suspected. Infectious epididymitis has a similar appearance. (*Courtesy of Richard E. Berger, M.D.*)

SUGGESTED READING

Geisler WM, Krieger JN. Epididymitis. Chapter 60 in KK Holmes, et al., eds. *Sexually Transmitted Diseases.* 4th ed. New York, NY: McGraw-Hill; 2008:1127-46. *A comprehensive review in the premier STD text, with emphasis on sexually transmitted epididymitis.*

Tracy CR, et al. Diagnosis and management of epididymitis. *Urol Clin N Am.* 2008;35:101-8. *A clinically oriented review.*

17

Reactive Arthritis

Reactive arthritis* is classically described as a triad of rheumatoid factor–negative arthritis, urethritis or cervicitis, and mucocutaneous inflammatory lesions, including conjunctivitis and a characteristic dermatitis. The syndrome results from an aberrant immune response after an initial triggering event, including genital infection with *Chlamydia trachomatis* and perhaps *Neisseria gonorrhoeae*, as well as enteric pathogens, including *Salmonella*, *Shigella*, *Campylobacter*, and *Yersinia*. In addition to the roles of chlamydial urethritis and cervicitis as triggering events, nongonococcal urethritis (NGU) and mucopurulent cervicitis are common manifestations of reactive arthritis, presumably due to an immunologic mechanism. Limited forms of the syndrome, such as isolated arthritis, are common at presentation, but most patients eventually develop mucocutaneous or ocular manifestations.

Reactive arthritis is clinically and pathologically related to other spondyloarthropathies like ankylosing spondylitis and psoriatic arthritis. Up to 90% of affected persons have the histocompatibility locus A (HLA) B27 haplotype. Reports of *C. trachomatis* antigens, DNA, and occasionally viable organisms in synovial tissues suggest a role of direct dissemination of the triggering infection in the pathogenesis of reactive arthritis, or in sustaining chronic arthritis in some patients. A proposed new terminology defines "*Chlamydia*-induced spondyloarthropathy" as a specific subset of reactive arthritis. In further support of persistent infection in pathogenesis, recent research suggests that a 6-month course of combination antibiotics (azithromycin or doxycycline, plus rifampin) helps control symptoms in patients with chronic forms of the syndrome.

Sporadically occurring reactive arthritis usually is triggered by genital infection, most frequently chlamydial NGU or cervicitis. Gonorrhea probably triggers some cases, which may present as "postgonococcal arthritis" and is distinct from the arthritis of disseminated gonococcal infection. Overt epidemics of reactive arthritis have occurred in populations with especially high prevalences of the HLA-B27 haplotype, as in Scandinavia, sometimes following outbreaks of enteric infection such as shigellosis or *Yersinia* enteritis.

---

*The former name, Reiter syndrome, is no longer used in light of revelations of Hans Reiter's human rights record, which included heinous human experimentation in concentration camp inmates during World War II.

Differentiating reactive arthritis from gonococcal arthritis is sometimes difficult, especially in sexually active persons who lack the characteristic skin lesions of either syndrome. Reactive arthritis usually is transient or causes modest functional limitation, but sometimes becomes disabling due to prolonged severe arthritis, secondary amyloidosis, or other complications.

EPIDEMIOLOGY

Incidence and Prevalence

- Among the most common causes of arthritis in young adults, but accurate statistics not available

Transmission

- Depends on triggering infection
- Person-to-person transmission of *Chlamydia*-linked reactive arthritis has been reported

Age

- All ages are susceptible
- Most cases occur in sexually active age groups
- Cases triggered by enteric infections have occurred in children as well as adults

Sex

- Modest male predominance, with male-female ratio 1:1 to 2:1
- Previously reported male-female ratios as high as 10:1 probably were due to reporting bias or under-diagnosis of cervicitis in women with seronegative arthritis

Sexual Orientation

- No special predilection
- MSM may be at increased risk due to elevated frequency of sexually acquired enteric infections

Other Risk Factors

- Frequency of reactive arthritis has been reported to be 20–35% following chlamydial or enteric infection in persons with HLA-B27 haplotype
- HIV-infected persons may be at elevated risk

HISTORY

Incubation Period

- Typically 1–4 weeks after onset of trigger infection

Symptoms

- Pain, swelling, and limited mobility of involved joints
  - Usually 1–3 joints involved in initial episode
  - Most commonly involved sites are heel, toes, lumbosacral spine, knee, or ankle, but any joint can be affected

- Symptoms of urethritis or cervicitis often are present

- Sometimes recent diarrhea or other symptoms of enteric infection

- Fever and other systemic symptoms may occur but usually are mild or absent

- Skin rash, symptoms of conjunctivitis, and oral ulcers (usually painless) may develop early or late

PHYSICAL EXAMINATION

Trigger Infection

- Signs of urethritis, cervicitis, or gastrointestinal infection (see Chaps. 15, 18, 21)

Arthritis

- Inflammatory signs of one or more joints

- Synovial effusion may be present when large joints are involved (e.g., knee, ankle)

- Tenderness often maximal at tendon insertion sites (entheses) (hence the rheumatologic classification of reactive arthritis as an "enthesopathy")

- Diffuse synovitis of one or more fingers or toes ("sausage digit") is uncommon but considered highly specific for reactive arthritis

- Sacroiliac joint tenderness may be present

Mucocutaneous Lesions

- Keratoderma blennorrhagica
  - Hyperkeratotic lesions with erythematous base, usually on extremities, sometimes in clusters
  - Resembles psoriasis clinically and histologically
  - Often involves palms and soles
  - May mimic secondary syphilis
  - Pustular component sometimes present

- Circinate balanitis: Superficially erosive dermatitis of the glans penis in uncircumcised men, often with a "geographic" morphology, is pathognomonic

- Conjunctivitis often present, usually bilateral

- Sometimes superficial ulcers of oral mucosa

Other Manifestations

- Fever, malaise, other constitutional symptoms; usually limited to severe cases

- Uncommon findings (<1% of cases) include iritis, uveitis, heart block or other cardiac arrhythmias, and focal neurological signs

- Amyloidosis is a rare complication of chronic cases

LABORATORY EVALUATION

- No definitive laboratory test exists

- Evaluate as for NGU and cervicitis (see Chaps. 15, 18), including NAATs for *C. trachomatis* and *N. gonorrhoeae*

- If synovial effusion present, aspirate for bacterial culture, leukocyte count, and analysis for crystals
- Blood cultures for to evaluate for bacterial septic arthritis, including gonococcal arthritis
- If current or gastrointestinal manifestations, test stool for enteric pathogens
- Serum rheumatoid factor test
- Erythrocyte sedimentation rate (ESR) or C-reactive protein (CRP) may be useful to follow clinical course and response to therapy
- HLA typing may help confirm diagnosis
- Several weeks after onset, x-ray lumbosacral spine; many patients develop radiological signs of sacroiliitis, whether or not there are symptoms of spinal involvement

DIAGNOSTIC CRITERIA

- American Rheumatism Association definition of reactive arthritis: Rheumatoid factor–negative arthritis >1 month in duration, associated with urethritis or cervicitis
- Exclude other causes of arthropathy, especially septic arthritis, DGI, and gout and other crystal-induced arthritis
- Synovial fluid usually has high cell count (>20,000/mm^3) with predominant PMNs
- HLA-B27 haplotype helps confirm diagnosis
- If DGI or septic arthritis cannot be excluded, consider therapeutic trial with IV antibiotics

TREATMENT

- Treat trigger infection with appropriate antibiotic, such as azithromycin or doxycycline for chlamydial infection or NGU (see Chaps. 3, 15)
- Mainstay of arthritis therapy is nonsteroidal anti-inflammatory drugs; aspirin and corticosteroids usually are ineffective
- Biological agents such as infliximab or adalumimab may have a role in management of chronic, disabling cases
- Azithromycin or doxycycline, plus rifampin, for 6 months may result in clinical improvement in some patients with chronic, disabling reactive arthritis; confirmatory research necessary
- Manage in consultation with a rheumatologist or other expert

PREVENTION

- Manage sex partners and report cases as dictated by triggering infection

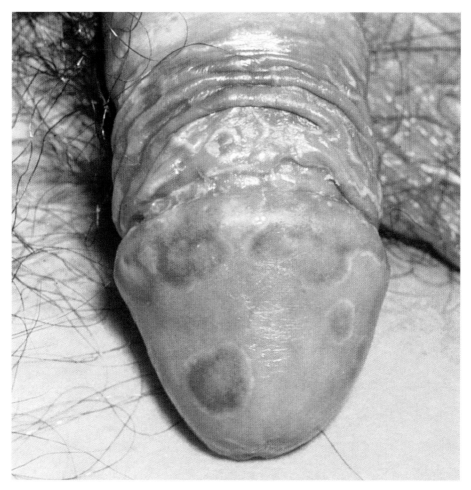

17–1. Reactive arthritis: circinate balanitis. *(Reprinted with permission from Holmes KK, et al, eds. Sexually Transmitted Diseases. 3rd ed. New York, NY: McGraw-Hill; 1999.)*

CASE

Patient Profile Age 27, surgery resident

History Low back pain and intermittent pain in both heels for 4 weeks; rash involving penis and feet for 3 days; pain and swelling of right knee for 1 day; no genital symptoms, diarrhea, fever, or other symptoms; last sexual exposure 2 months earlier

Examination Effusion and reduced range of motion of right knee; tenderness at Achilles tendon insertion sites of both heels; geographic eruption of glans penis and underside of foreskin; hyperkeratotic inflammatory skin lesions of lower extremities; no urethral discharge; 50 mL of cloudy synovial fluid aspirated from knee

Differential Diagnosis Reactive arthritis, psoriatic arthritis, ankylosing spondylitis, rheumatoid arthritis, disseminated gonococcal infection

Laboratory Gram-stained urethral smear showed many PMNs without GND; urethral swabs were cultured for *C. trachomatis* (positive) and *N. gonorrhoeae* (negative); synovial fluid contained 42,000 leukocytes per mm^3 with 90% PMNs, no crystals, negative Gram stain and culture; rheumatoid factor and VDRL negative; complete blood count and chemistry panel normal; ESR 43 mm/h; HLA-B27 positive

Diagnosis Reactive arthritis triggered by *C. trachomatis*

Treatment Doxycycline 100 mg orally *bid* for 7 days; indomethacin 150 mg orally *tid*

Partner Management Referred for examination and treatment for chlamydial infection

Comment The patient had prompt symptomatic response, permitting cessation of indomethacin after 2 months. His most recent sex partner was referred, found to have cervical chlamydia, and treated. Subsequently he had persistent but nonlimiting low back pain, and sacroiliac radiographs after 1 year showed hypertrophic changes and narrowed joint spaces. Currently, naproxen or other nonsteroidal anti-inflammatory drug would normally be used in lieu of indomethacin.

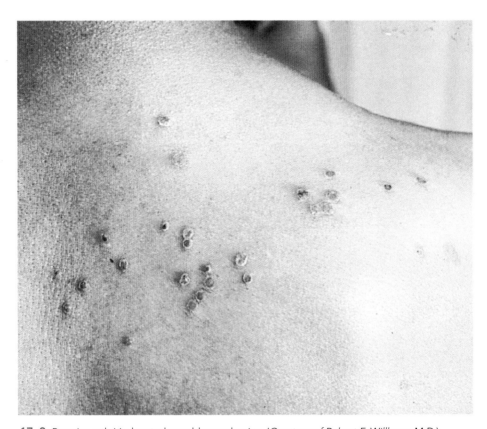

17–2. Reactive arthritis: keratoderma blennorrhagica. (*Courtesy of Robert F. Willkens, M.D.*)

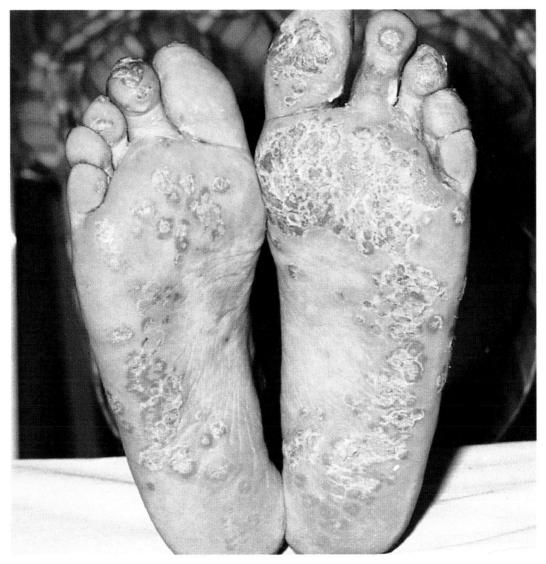

17–3. Severe plantar keratoderma blennorrhagica in chronic reactive arthritis. Compare with secondary syphilis (see Fig. 5–16). (*Courtesy of Robert F. Willkens, M.D.*)

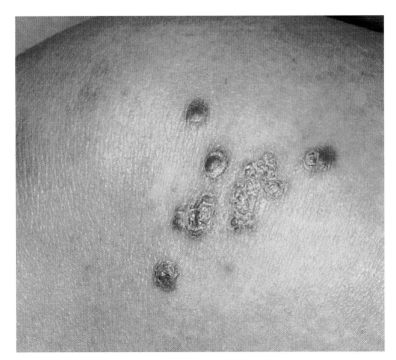

17–4. Cutaneous lesions of the knee consistent with keratoderma blennorrhagica or psoriasis in a woman with acute spondyloarthritis. The patient was the sex partner of a man with NGU, but lacked evidence of *C. trachomatis*, cervicitis, or other lower genital tract infection and was HLA-B27 positive. Reactive arthritis and psoriatic arthritis could not be differentiated.

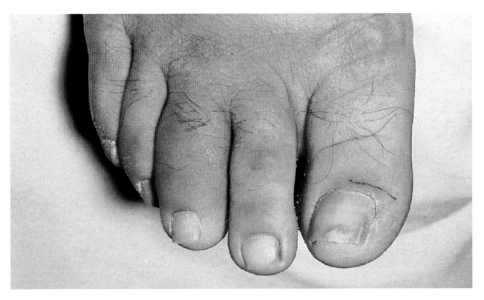

17–5. Diffuse dactylitis ("sausage toe") of third digit in a patient with reactive arthritis. (*Courtesy of Robert F. Willkens, M.D.*)

SUGGESTED READING

Carter JD, Hudson AP. Reactive arthritis: clinical aspects and medical management. *Rheum Dis Clin North Am.* 2009;35:21-44. *An up-to-date clinical review by two leading investigators of reactive arthritis.*

Rice PA, Handsfield HH. Arthritis associated with sexually transmitted diseases. Chapter 67 in KK Holmes, et al., eds. *Sexually Transmitted Diseases.* 4th ed. New York, NY: McGraw-Hill; 2008:1259-76. *A comprehensive review of STD-related arthritis syndromes, in the premier STD textbook.*

Rihl M, et al. Combination antibiotics for *Chlamydia*-induced arthritis: breakthrough to a cure? *Arth Rheum.* 2010;1203-7. *An editorial and review of controversies in pathogenesis and treatment of chronic Chlamydia-associated reactive arthritis, in response to a research report in the same issue (Arth Rheum 2010;1298-307) that documented clinical improvement in response to 6-month regimens of azithromycin or doxycycline, plus rifampin.*

18

Mucopurulent Cervicitis

Mucopurulent cervicitis (MPC) is characterized by inflammation of the endocervical mucosa and is generally regarded as the female counterpart of urethritis in men. The major defined causes are *Chlamydia trachomatis* and *Neisseria gonorrhoeae*, but in common usage MPC usually implies chlamydial or other nongonococcal infection. *Mycoplasma genitalium* may cause some cases. Herpes simplex virus (HSV) and *Trichomonas vaginalis* can cause MPC as well, usually in conjunction with ectocervicitis. Bacterial vaginosis (BV) is associated with MPC, but the causal relationship is uncertain. As for urethritis in men, the cause of MPC remains obscure for at least half of the cases. Accurate diagnosis of MPC can be difficult and strongly depends on provider training and experience. Some signs, such as edematous cervical ectopy and purulence of endocervical secretions, are subjective, especially for providers with limited clinical experience. Examination of Gram-stained endocervical secretions for semiquantitation of polymorphonuclear leukocytes has been used successfully to help define the syndrome for research purposes, but has been difficult to employ in clinical settings due to problems in standardization and frequent lack of ready access to microscopy.

Pelvic inflammatory disease is the primary recognized complication but is clearly linked only with MPC caused by chlamydial infection or gonorrhea. It is not known whether idiopathic MPC, without an identified pathogen, carries important health consequences for patients or their sex partners, and agreement is lacking on the need for antibiotic therapy in the absence of *C. trachomatis*, *N. gonorrhoeae*, and *M. genitalium*. Treatment with azithromycin or doxycycline is indicated while awaiting the results of diagnostic tests for gonorrhea and chlamydia, especially in younger women. Patients with idiopathic MPC that persists after one or two courses of antibiotic therapy should be evaluated for associated infections such as herpes, trichomoniasis, and BV. If cervicitis persists after these have been excluded or treated, repeated courses of antibiotics are unlikely to be beneficial.

EPIDEMIOLOGY

Incidence and Prevalence

- Accurate statistics not available
- Present in 10–20% of women in most STD clinics, but highly variable, due in part to varying clinical recognition

Transmission

- As for gonorrhea and chlamydial infection (see Chaps. 3 and 4)
- No data exist on transmission frequency and risks for etiologically undefined MPC
- Uncommon in sexually inactive women, implying sexual acquisition or association with intercourse

Age

- Most common in teens, in whom physiologic cervical ectopy may predispose to *C. trachomatis* and other inflammatory factors
- MPC in women ≤25 years old is especially likely to be due to chlamydial infection or gonorrhea

Other Risk Factors

- Cervical ectopy, i.e., endocervical columnar mucosa extending onto ectocervix
  - Ectopy is normal in adolescence and is a physiologic response to hormonal influences (e.g., pregnancy, oral contraceptives)
  - Physiologic ectopy may increase infection risk by exposing susceptible epithelium
  - Transient ectopy can result from cervical edema due to inflammation, causing eversion that exposes endocervical mucosa
- Pregnancy and hormonal contraception appear to increase risk of MPC

HISTORY

Incubation Period

- Uncertain; probably usually 1–4 weeks, as for chlamydia and gonorrhea

Symptoms

- Most cases asymptomatic
- Increased vaginal discharge
- Intermenstrual bleeding, often manifested as postcoital bleeding
- Dysuria may be present due to concomitant urethritis
- Genital malodor absent except in cases associated with BV or trichomoniasis

Epidemiologic History

- STD risk factors usually present
- Especially common in sexually active teens

PHYSICAL EXAMINATION

- Mucopurulent exudate emanating from cervical os
- Purulence (yellow color) of cervical secretions; best assessed on swab examined outside vagina ("swab test")
- Edematous ectopy of exposed endocervical mucosa

- Endocervical bleeding induced by gentle swabbing (sometimes called "friability")
- Mild cervical tenderness may be found on bimanual pelvic examination

LABORATORY EVALUATION

- NAATs for *C. trachomatis* and *N. gonorrhoeae* (see Chaps. 3 and 4)
- Examine and test vaginal secretions for *T. vaginalis* (by NAAT, if available), BV, and yeasts (see Chap. 19)
- NAAT or culture for HSV if:
  - Ectocervicitis or ulceration (see Chap. 8)
  - Mucocutaneous vesicles, pustules, or ulcers
  - HSV exposure history

DIAGNOSIS

The diagnosis of MPC can be considered firm in presence of two or more of the following criteria. Presumptive therapy for gonorrhea and chlamydial infection may be warranted in presence of only one criterion, especially in women <25 years old.

- Mucopurulent cervical exudate, by direct visualization or positive "swab test"
- Edematous cervical ectopy
- Swab-induced endocervical bleeding
- Gram-stained endocervical smear showing increased PMNs, often within strands of mucus

MANAGEMENT

Treatment

- Treat as for uncomplicated chlamydial infection (see Chap. 3)
  - Azithromycin 1.0 g PO (single dose); *or*
  - Doxycycline 100 mg PO *bid* for 7 days
- Also give treatment for gonorrhea in patients and settings at high risk for gonococcal infection (see Chap. 4)
  - Ceftriaxone 250 mg IM, single dose; *or*
  - Cefixime 400 mg PO, single dose
- Physical ablation of cervical mucosa (e.g., cryotherapy, laser cautery) sometimes is attempted for persistent, antibiotic-resistant MPC, but efficacy is unknown and such measures are generally not recommended

Partner Management

- Male partners should be evaluated and treated presumptively for chlamydia, and for gonorrhea if indicated by risk profile
- EPT has not been studied except for confirmed gonorrhea or chlamydia, but is an option when partners are unlikely to attend for professional care (see Chaps. 1, 3, and 4)
- Treatment generally is not recommended for partners of patients with MPC that persists after antibiotic treatment

Follow-up

- As for chlamydial infection or gonorrhea (see Chaps. 3 and 4)
- Clinical follow-up usually not required unless symptoms persist

PARTNER MANAGEMENT AND PREVENTION

- Depending on suspected or documented cause, manage partners as described for gonorrhea, chlamydial infection, or NGU (*See Chaps. 3, 4, and 15*).
- General STD prevention measures (partner selection, condoms) presumably reduce risk of MPC

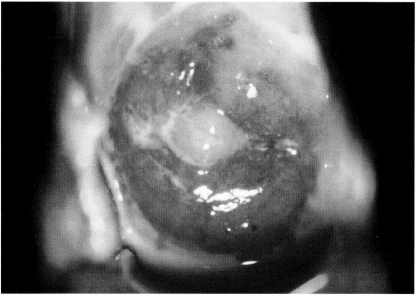

a

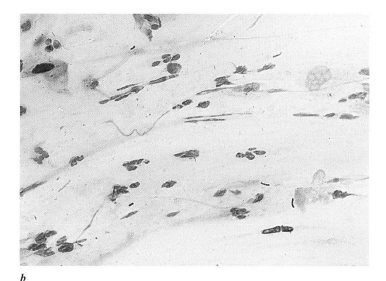

b

18–1. Mucopurulent cervicitis. *a.* Edematous cervical ectopy and mucopurulent exudate in cervical os. *b.* Gram-stained smear of endocervical secretions, showing PMNs in mucus strands; a few lactobacilli but no gram-negative diplococci are present. Mucus indicates endocervical origin of secretions, because vaginal mucosa lacks mucus glands.

CASE

Patient Profile Age 16, high school student

History Slight increased vaginal discharge for 10 days; responded to partner notification after her boyfriend was diagnosed with NGU

Examination External genitals normal; cervix showed edematous ectopy, mucopurulent exudate in os

Differential Diagnosis MPC, probably due to *C. trachomatis*; possible gonorrhea, trichomoniasis, herpes

Laboratory Gram-stained endocervical smear showed numerous PMNs in mucus strands, without gram-negative diplococci (GND); vaginal fluid pH 4.0; negative KOH amine odor test; no yeasts, clue cells, or trichomonads seen on wet-mount microscopy; cervical NAATs for *C. trachomatis* (positive) and *N. gonorrhoeae* (negative); RPR and HIV serology (both negative)

Diagnosis MPC due to *C. trachomatis*

Treatment Azithromycin 1.0 g PO, single dose

Comment This patient presented with typical chlamydial MPC and would have qualified for presumptive treatment for chlamydial infection regardless of exposure to infected partner.

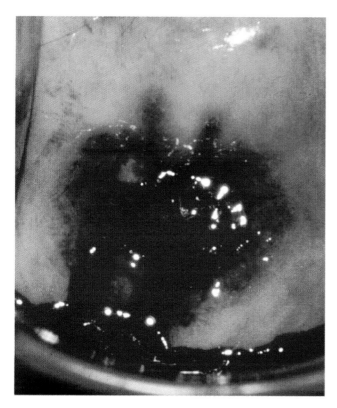

18–2. Mucopurulent cervicitis; bleeding induced by endocervical swab. (*Courtesy of Claire E. Stevens.*)

CASE

Patient Profile Age 33, clerk-receptionist

History Intermittent increased vaginal discharge without abnormal odor; married for 5 years, no extramarital partners; several years' history of intermittent, unexplained vaginal discharge, postcoital blood spotting, and Pap smears with inflammatory changes, unresponsive to previous courses of antibiotics and cervical cryotherapy; patient presented to STD clinic to "make sure once and for all" that no STD was present

Examination External genitals normal; cervix showed mucopurulent exudate in os and brisk endocervical bleeding induced by swabs used to collect culture specimens

Differential Diagnosis Mucopurulent cervicitis; rule out gonorrhea, chlamydial infection, trichomoniasis, herpes

Laboratory Endocervical smear showed many PMNs, no GND; vaginal fluid pH 4.5 with negative KOH amine odor test; no yeasts, clue cells, or trichomonads seen microscopically on wet mount; cervical NAATs for *C. trachomatis* and *N. gonorrhoeae* (both negative); cultures for *T. vaginalis* and HSV (both negative); VDRL, HIV, HSV-1, and HSV-2 serology (all negative); Pap smear showed inflammation, otherwise normal and negative for HPV DNA

Diagnosis Idiopathic (apparently persistent or recurrent) MPC

Comment Treatment was deferred at the patient's initial visit, because both medical history and patient's age made chlamydial infection and gonorrhea unlikely. She returned after 1 week with persistent symptoms and unchanged examination. Her husband denied other sex partners, was examined and found to have no evidence of urethritis, and had negative tests for *C. trachomatis* and *N. gonorrhoeae*. Both were treated with doxycycline 100 mg PO *bid* for 7 days. The patient's symptoms persisted on therapy, then improved over the next 2 months, but repeat examination was unchanged. The patient was seen several years ago; current management would include NAAT for *M. genitalium* if available, treatment with azithromycin, and trial of metronidazole or tinidazole for possible trichomoniasis. The patient and her husband were reassured that no long-term adverse consequences were expected

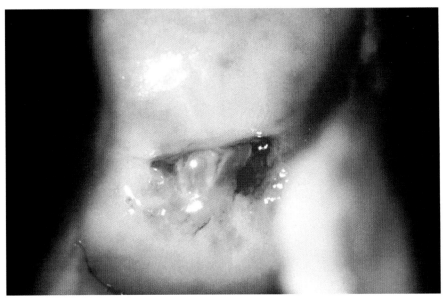

a

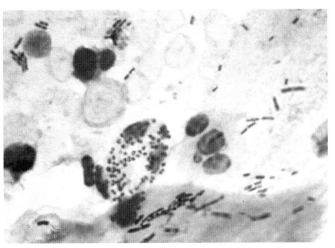

b

18–3. Mucopurulent cervicitis due to *N. gonorrhoeae*. *a*. Mucopurulent endocervical exudate. Note that the purulence of cervical exudate does not correlate well with gonococcal or non-gonococcal etiology, unlike urethritis in men. *b*. Gram-stained endocervical smear, showing a single PMN with ICGND. (*Courtesy of Claire E. Stevens.*)

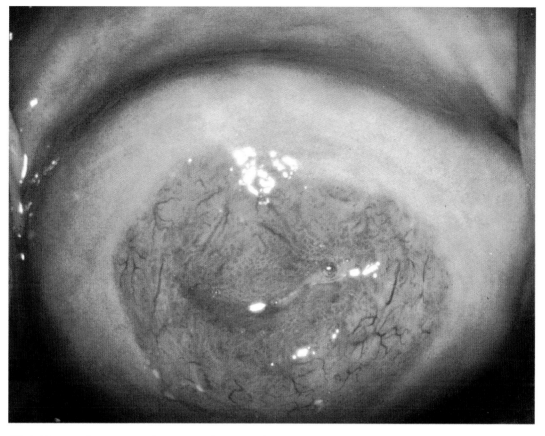

18–4. Mucopurulent cervicitis due to *C. trachomatis*; edematous cervical ectopy and scant mucoid exudate. (*Courtesy of Claire E. Stevens.*)

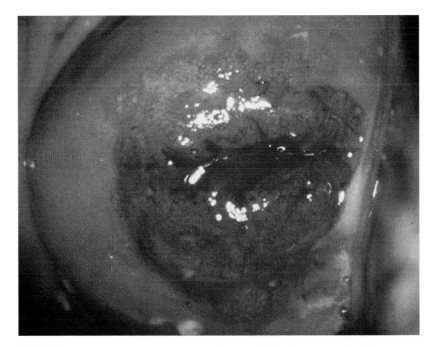

18–5. Edematous ectopy with incipient endocervical bleeding in a patient with mucopurulent cervicitis; her chief complaint was postcoital bleeding. (*Courtesy of Claire E. Stevens.*)

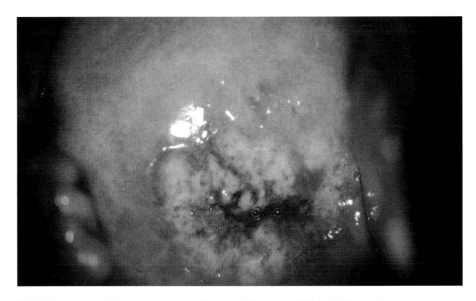

18–6. Erosive cervicitis in primary genital herpes. (*Courtesy of Claire E. Stevens.*)

SUGGESTED READING

Brunham RC, et al. Mucopurulent cervicitis: the ignored counterpart in women of urethritis in men. *N Engl J Med.* 1984;311:1-6. *The first systematic description of the clinical syndrome and etiology of MPC, still clinically applicable.*

Holmes KK, Stamm WE, Sobel JE. Lower genital tract infection syndromes in women. Chapter 55 in KK Holmes, et al., eds. *Sexually Transmitted Diseases.* 4th ed. New York, NY: McGraw-Hill; 2008:987-1016. *An authoritative, comprehensive, extensively referenced review of cervical, urethral, and vaginal infections in women.*

Marrazzo JM, Martin DH. Management of women with cervicitis. *Clin Infect Dis.* 2007;44(Suppl 3):S102-10. *Review of the data in support of CDC's 2006 STD treatment guidelines.*

Wilson JF. In the clinic: vaginitis and cervicitis. *Ann Intern Med.* 2009;151:ITIC3 1-15. *A comprehensive, well-referenced review of clinical aspects, with a combined syndromic and etiologic approach.*

19

Vaginal Infections

Vulvovaginal yeast infections, bacterial vaginosis, and trichomoniasis are among the most common reasons for which women seek health care in the United States and probably in other industrialized countries. All sexually active women with trichomoniasis or new onset of bacterial vaginosis, and many with candidiasis, should be evaluated for other common STDs.

Vulvovaginal Candidiasis

Vulvovaginal candidiasis (VVC) generally is not sexually transmitted and most symptomatic episodes do not result from exogenous infection. Rather, *Candida albicans* and sometimes *C. glabrata* are normal commensal flora of the vagina and colon, and clinically evident VVC results when known factors (e.g., suppression of vaginal bacterial flora by antibiotics, hyperglycemia in diabetes) and unknown ones result in proliferation of yeasts or development of an allergic response to them. A small minority of infections may be acquired from sex partners with genital or oral colonization with *Candida*. Symptomatic VVC typically is accompanied by external genital symptoms and signs (vulvitis), yet vaginal fluid leukocytosis usually is absent.

Uncomplicated VVC is defined as sporadic, infrequent cases of mild or moderate severity in immunocompetent women who are likely to be infected with *C. albicans*. Complicated VVC includes recurrent infections, clinically severe cases, infection with *C. glabrata*, and VVC in immunocompromised women or those with uncontrolled diabetes, and requires more intensive or more prolonged treatment and may warrant ongoing prophylactic therapy. Single-dose oral treatment with fluconazole is effective against uncomplicated VVC and often is preferred by patients over intravaginal therapy. Effective vaginal preparations for treatment of VVC are available over the counter. However, self-treatment for vaginal discharge risks delayed diagnosis of STDs, and should be restricted to patients with previous professionally diagnosed VVC who have typical recurrent symptoms.

Bacterial Vaginosis

Bacterial vaginosis (BV) is characterized by overgrowth of commensal vaginal bacteria, including *Gardnerella vaginalis, Mobiluncus* species, *Prevotella* species, *Mycoplasma hominis*, and numerous anaerobes. Hydrogen peroxide-producing *Lactobacillus crispatus* and other lactobacilli, which maintain an aerobic, acidic milieu in the healthy vagina, are absent in BV or present in greatly reduced amounts. One hypothesis of pathogenesis is that failure of *Lactobacillus* colonization is the initiating event in BV, but the specific causes are unknown. Novel bacterial vaginosis-associated bacteria types 1, 2, and 3 (BVAB-1, -2, and -3) have been identified by 16s ribosomal analysis but not yet cultured. They appear to be specifically associated with the syndrome, but it remains uncertain whether BVAB have a direct etiologic role in BV. There is little or no inflammatory response in BV and leukocytes usually are not found in vaginal fluid, hence the term *vaginosis*, not vaginitis.

Bacterial vaginosis is associated with sexual intercourse and with the same epidemiologic markers as classical STDs, such as multiple sex partners, new partners, and past history of STDs, but whether BV should be classified as an STD is controversial. Direct sexual transmission clearly occurs in women who have sex with women, through shared vaginal secretions, and almost all female sex partners of women with BV have the syndrome themselves. It has been reported that BV can occur in sexually inexperienced women, i.e., without history of penile-vaginal intercourse. However, recent studies show the syndrome to occur rarely if ever in women who have had no vaginal sexual exposures, including cunnilingus, suggesting that the initial occurrence of BV may require exogenous infection with a sexually transmitted pathogen. On the other hand, no recognized sexually transmitted organism has been directly linked with BV, and treatment of women's male partners does not apparently influence the rate of recurrence following treatment, although it is uncertain whether optimal therapies have been employed. Whether or not BV is an STD in the usual sense, affected women are at elevated risk for other STDs, and routine screening and STD prevention counseling are indicated for women with the syndrome.

Bacterial vaginosis is associated with elevated risks of pelvic inflammatory disease (PID), premature labor, and other complications of labor and delivery, but in a large randomized controlled trial the frequency of adverse pregnancy outcomes was not reduced by treatment of BV in pregnant women. Many women with BV attempt self-treatment with vaginal douching, but vaginal douching itself predisposes to BV and is epidemiologically linked with PID and ectopic pregnancy. Clinicians should discourage women from douching for any reason, including vulvovaginal "hygiene," odor, discharge, or following menstruation or intercourse. Treatment of BV is based primarily on anti-anaerobic antibiotics, ideally with drugs like metronidazole that do not inhibit *Lactobacillus*, which might retard repopulation of the vagina with protective biota.

Trichomoniasis

Trichomoniasis is a common sexually transmitted infection caused by the unicellular parasite *Trichomonas vaginalis*. Apparent exceptions to sexual transmission generally are explained by delayed diagnosis of longstanding infection, or by acquisition from chronically infected sex partners. Symptomatic trichomoniasis is associated with an inflammatory response and vaginal leukocytosis and is accompanied by anaerobic bacterial overgrowth and depletion of lactobacilli, as in BV. Other STDs, such as gonorrhea or chlamydial infection, often are present. Infected men usually are asymptomatic, but some have nongonococcal urethritis (NGU), and *T. vaginalis* can be identified by nucleic acid amplification test (NAAT) in about 5% of NGU cases. Heretofore widely considered a trivial infection, trichomoniasis is emerging as an important STD that causes significant morbidity in women both directly and through enhanced susceptibility to sexually transmitted HIV. Evidence is mounting that routine screening and other public health prevention measures are warranted, a case made stronger by development and increasing availability of *T. vaginalis* NAATs.

Single-dose treatment with oral metronidazole is the usual therapy, but is only about 90% effective; multiple-dose regimens are more reliable. Tinidazole, a related drug, is more expensive than metronidazole but perhaps more effective, especially in single doses and in men. Intravaginal metronidazole is ineffective. Occasional strains of *T. vaginalis* are resistant to both drugs, making treatment difficult. High-dose intravenous metronidazole sometimes is effective, and case reports suggest that intravaginal therapy with paromomycin or furazolidone may be useful options.

Other Vulvovaginal Syndromes

Uncommon causes of vulvovaginal infection or increased vaginal discharge include retained foreign bodies (e.g., tampons), enterovaginal fistulas, and estrogen deficiency. Physiologic leucorrhea, i.e., fluctuations in the quantity or character of cervicovaginal secretions, explains some women's complaints of increased vaginal discharge. Idiopathic vulvodynia and desquamative inflammatory vaginitis are vexing clinical problems that are not attributable to any known STD.

EPIDEMIOLOGY

Incidence and Prevalence

- Among women attending STD or reproductive health clinics, VVC is diagnosed in 20–25%, BV in 10–20%, trichomoniasis in 5–15%
- Most women age 15–40 years experience one or more episodes of VVC
- In a population-based U.S. sample (NHANES) 2001–2004, 3.2% of women had trichomoniasis and 33% had BV

Transmission

- Vaginal colonization with *Candida* species is present in 10–20% of healthy women of reproductive age, often originating from colonic reservoir
- Transmission of BV uncertain
  - Associated with sexual activity, but sexual transmission between males and females remains uncertain
  - Directly transmitted between female sex partners through shared vaginal secretions
- *T. vaginalis* is sexually transmitted and acquired

Age

- No particular predilection
- All three syndromes are most frequent in young women

Sex

- BV has no known male counterpart
- Male partners of women with VVC sometimes have penile *Candida* dermatitis or balanitis

- *T. vaginalis* colonizes male urethra and periurethral glands
  - Usually asymptomatic
  - Accounts for ~5% of NGU

Sexual Orientation

- BV is common in WSW; female sex partners of women with BV almost invariably have BV themselves
- WSW are not apparently at either increased or reduced risk for VVC or trichomoniasis, but few data available

Other Risk Factors

- Douching increases risk of BV, probably by disrupting normal vaginal ecology
- Diaphragm, contraceptive sponge, and nonoxynol-9–based spermicides apparently predispose to BV and perhaps VVC
- Antibiotic therapy predisposes to VVC and perhaps BV
- Poorly controlled diabetes mellitus predisposes to vaginal colonization with *Candida* and VVC, sometimes severe
- Except for overt AIDS, HIV infection is not associated with substantially enhanced risk of VVC, despite earlier reports to the contrary; however, HIV infection may impair response of VVC to treatment
- Tight-fitting garments probably do not predispose to VVC, notwithstanding common beliefs

HISTORY

Incubation Period

- VVC usually is not attributable to exogenous infection with *Candida* species; occurs in previously colonized women as result of enhanced growth of *Candida* or allergic reaction to it
- Symptoms of trichomoniasis or BV often begin a few days to 4 weeks after sexual exposure to new or infected partners

Symptoms

Vulvovaginal Candidiasis

- Vulvar burning pain or pruritus
- "External" dysuria from contact of urine with inflamed introitus and labia
- Vaginal discharge usually absent or scant
- Usually no malodor (contrary to popular belief)

Bacterial Vaginosis

- Genital malodor, often described as "fishy," is the most common symptom
- Odor may be more prominent following intercourse; alkalinity of semen volatilizes amine products of anaerobic bacterial metabolism

- Increased vaginal discharge
  - Inflammatory response and leukocytes are usually absent; therefore discharge does not cause prominent staining of underclothes
- Often asymptomatic

Trichomoniasis

- Increased vaginal discharge, often profuse
  - Staining of underclothes (secretions are inflammatory with elevated leukocytes)
- Malodor, often "fishy"; sometimes prominent after vaginal intercourse (See Bacterial Vaginosis)
- Vulvar pruritus
- Most prevalent cases are asymptomatic

Epidemiologic History

- Risk factors for STD often are present in women with BV or trichomoniasis
- STD risk is not associated with VVC
- Antibiotic use precedes some VVC and BV
- Women with BV or VVC often give history of prior episodes

PHYSICAL EXAMINATION

Vulvovaginal Candidiasis

- Vulvar erythema, sometimes with edema or superficial fissures
- Typical discharge is scant, clumped, white, adherent to vaginal mucosa, but appearance is quite variable and can include flocculent or purulent-appearing exudate
- Complicated or severe VVC: Vulvar erythema or edema, often with superficial fissures and excoriation

Bacterial Vaginosis

- Discharge typically white, homogeneous, smoothly coating vaginal walls or labia; scant to moderate in amount
- Usually no erythema or other inflammatory signs
- Signs of MPC may be present (see Chap. 18)

Trichomoniasis

- Discharge typically copious and purulent (creamy, yellow, or brown)
- Bubbles in vaginal fluid are said to be highly specific for trichomoniasis, but usually absent
- Mucosal erythema may be present
- Cervix may show signs of MPC (see Chap.18)
- Occasional petechiae on ectocervix ("colpitis macularis," "strawberry cervix")

DIAGNOSTIC APPROACH

The first step in evaluating a woman with increased vaginal discharge or other vulvovaginal complaints is a speculum examination to determine whether abnormal secretions originate from the vagina or cervix. The character of the vaginal discharge is assessed and the vaginal mucosa and vulva are inspected for erythema, edema, ulcers, and other lesions. Table 19-1 displays the usual characteristics of VVC, trichomoniasis, BV, and uninfected women. An accurate office diagnosis usually can be made by determination of the pH of vaginal secretions, testing for amine (fishy) odor on addition of 10% KOH, and microscopy of vaginal fluid by saline and KOH wet mounts, Gram stain, or all three. However, saline microscopy is only 60–70% sensitive for *T. vaginalis* in symptomatic trichomoniasis and probably is <50% sensitive in asymptomatically infected women. Culture for *T. vaginalis* improves sensitivity, but NAAT is now the test of choice and is increasingly available in clinical laboratories. Culture for yeasts also may be helpful when VVC is suspected but not confirmed microscopically, but positive cultures for *Candida* species must be interpreted with caution because many women are colonized without symptoms. Rapid, office-based chemical tests for BV flora or chemical markers may also be useful; a rapid test for sialidase, a product of anaerobic metabolism, is in wide use. Screening tests for chlamydial infection, gonorrhea, syphilis, and HIV infection should be routine in all women with trichomoniasis or initial episodes of BV, and in selected women with VVC or recurrent BV, depending on sexual history.

LABORATORY DIAGNOSIS

Vulvovaginal Candidiasis

- Vaginal fluid pH ≤4.5

- Negative amine odor with 10% KOH

- Vaginal fluid microscopy (Gram-stained smear or saline mount) demonstrates pseudohyphae or yeasts in ~80% of patients; visualization of fungal elements may be aided by KOH wet mount, which digests cells and highlights yeasts and pseudohyphae

- PMNs usually absent or scant

- Visualization of yeasts alone (without pseudohyphae) is not diagnostic; may indicate asymptomatic colonization

- Isolation of *Candida* species may be helpful if microscopy is negative, but may be positive due to asymptomatic colonization

Bacterial Vaginosis

- Vaginal fluid pH > 4.5 (usually ≥4.7)

- Amine odor with 10% KOH (liberates volatile amines produced by anaerobic bacteria)

- Saline mount or Gram-stained smear showing clue cells, i.e., epithelial cells with granular appearance and indistinct borders due to adherent bacteria

- PMNs usually absent

- Gram stain shows profusion of mixed gram-positive and gram-negative bacteria, and absence of Gram-positive bacilli typical of *Lactobacillus* species

- Test for sialidase, liberated by vaginal bacteria in BV, (e.g., BVblue) may be a useful diagnostic aid

TABLE 19–1 DIAGNOSTIC FEATURES OF VAGINAL INFECTION IN PREMENOPAUSAL WOMEN

	Normal	Vulvovaginal Candidiasis	Trichomoniasis	Bacterial Vaginosis
Typical symptoms	None, or no change in vaginal discharge	Vulvar itching and/or irritation; sometimes increased discharge	Purulent discharge, often profuse; malodor; sometimes vulvar pruritus	Vulvovaginal malodor; slightly increased discharge
Discharge Amount	Variable; usually scant	Scant to moderate	Profuse	Scant to moderate
Color*	Clear or white	White or yellow	Yellow, light brown	Usually white
Consistency	Nonhomogeneous, floccular	Clumped; adherent plaques	Homogeneous; occasionally with bubbles	Homogeneous, thin (i.e., low viscosity); smoothly coats vaginal mucosa
Epithelial or mucosal inflammation	None	Erythema of vaginal epithelium, introitus; vulvar erythema; fissures or excoriations in severe cases	Erythema of vaginal and vulvar epithelium; sometimes petechiae of ectocervix ("strawberry cervix")	Usually none
pH of vaginal fluid†	≤4.5	≤4.5	>4.5 (often >5.0)	>4.5
Amine (fishy) odor with 10% KOH	None	None	Present	Present
Microscopy‡	Normal epithelial cells; predominant large Gram-positive rods (lactobacilli)	Epithelial cells; yeasts or pseudomycelia (up to 80%); few or no PMNs	PMNs; motile trichomonads in 60–70% of symptomatic patients; clue cells and altered bacteria similar to BV	Clue cells; profuse mixed flora; few or no lactobacilli

*Color of discharge is determined by examination outside vagina in bright light against a white background.
†pH may be falsely elevated in presence of blood.
‡To detect fungal elements, vaginal fluid is digested with 10% KOH prior to microscopic examination; to examine for clue cells, leukocytes and trichomonads, fluid is mixed 1:1 with physiologic saline solution. Gram stain also is excellent for detecting yeasts and pseudomycelia and for distinguishing normal flora from the mixed flora seen in bacterial vaginosis, but is insensitive for detection of *T. vaginalis*.

Trichomoniasis

- Vaginal fluid pH >4.5 (usually ≥5.0)
- Motile trichomonads (60–70% sensitive) and predominant PMNs on saline microscopy of vaginal secretions
- NAAT or culture for *T. vaginalis* if trichomoniasis suspected and microscopy negative
- Clue cells and positive amine odor test usually present, as in BV

TREATMENT

Vulvovaginal Candidiasis
Uncomplicated VVC

- Fluconazole 150 mg PO (single dose)
- Intravaginal imidazole
  - Several creams or suppositories are available (butoconazole, clotrimazole, miconazole, terconazole, or tioconazole)
  - Administer once daily for 3–7 days (single-dose regimens not recommended)
  - Several are available over the counter
- Nystatin vaginal tablets 100,000 units once daily for 14 days

Complicated VVC

- Severe VVC or immunocompromised patient
  - Fluconazole 150 mg PO twice, 3 days apart; *or*
  - Vaginal imidazole for 7-14 days
  - Correct modifiable conditions (e.g., diabetes control)
- VVC caused by *C. glabrata* or other non-albicans species
  - Imidazole therapy other than fluconazole, e.g., a vaginal imidazole for 7-14 days
  - Boric acid in gelatin capsules, 600 mg vaginally once daily for 14 days
- Prevention of recurrent VVC
  - Fluconazole 150-200 mg PO once weekly; *or*
  - Vaginal imidazole or nystatin once weekly

Partner Management

- Routine referral of partners is not recommended
- Male partners with symptoms that suggest penile dermatitis may benefit from topical antifungal therapy

Bacterial Vaginosis

Vaginal douching should not be used and should be assertively discouraged for treatment or prevention of BV or for vaginal hygiene. Currently available *Lactobacillus* preparations and dairy products (e.g., yogurt) do not contain physiologic *Lactobacillus* strains that produce hydrogen peroxide, do not successfully colonize the vagina, and are ineffective for treatment or prophylaxis, whether used orally or intravaginally. Research is under way to develop therapeutic products based on *L. crispatus* or other human lactobacilli.

Treatments of Choice

- Metronidazole 500 mg PO *bid* for 7 days
- Metronidazole gel 0.75% 5 g intravaginally once daily for 5 days
- Clindamycin 2% cream 5 g intravaginally once daily at bedtime for 7 days

Alternatives

- Tinidazole 2.0 g PO once daily for 3 days
- Tinidazole 1.0 g PO once daily for 5 days
- Clindamycin 300 mg PO *bid* for 7 days
- Clindamycin vaginal ovules 100 mg intravaginally once daily at bedtime for 3 days

Follow-up

- Reevaluate after 1-2 weeks if symptoms persist

Partner Management

- Evaluate male partners of women with first-episode BV
- No treatment is recommended for male partners without evidence of STD
- Advise WSW that their female partners are likely to have BV

Trichomoniasis

Treatments of Choice

- Tinidazole 2.0 g PO, single dose
- Metronidazole 2.0 g PO, single dose

Alternative Treatments

Multiple-dose therapy is indicated whenever trichomoniasis persists or recurs after treatment of patient and sex partners.

- Tinidazole 500 mg PO *bid* for 5 days
- Metronidazole 500 mg PO *bid* for 7 days

Follow-up

- Both reinfection and treatment failure (with single-dose therapy) are common
- Reevaluate 1 week after treatment if symptoms persist
- Rescreen women for *T. vaginalis* 3 months after treatment, using NAAT or culture

Partner Management

- Evaluate partners for urethritis and other STD
- Treat routinely with tinidazole 2.0 g (single dose) or metronidazole 2.0 g PO (single dose)
- EPT has uncertain efficacy but is warranted if partner is unlikely to attend for care

PREVENTION

Vulvovaginal Candidiasis

- Manage predisposing causes (e.g., diabetes control)
- Avoid unnecessary antibiotic therapy
- Prophylactic antifungal therapy in patients with recurrent VVC

Bacterial Vaginosis

- Recurrent BV is common, vexing, and difficult to prevent
- Condoms may help prevent some episodes in women with recurrent BV
- Treatment of female partners may help prevent reinfection
- Avoid douching

Trichomoniasis

- Treatment of sex partners
- Routine STD prevention measures (partner selection, condoms, etc.)

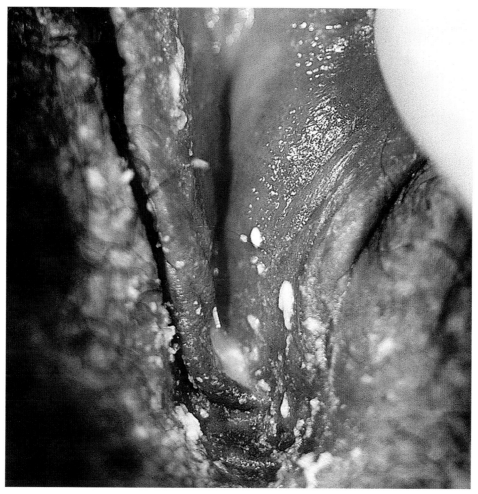

19–1. *Candida* vulvovaginitis; erythema and edema of labia minora and scant, clumped white exudate.

CASE

Patient Profile Age 20, university student, sexually active with one male partner

History Vulvar itching and slightly increased vaginal discharge for 2 days

Examination Faint erythema of vaginal introitus and labia minor; plaques of clumped white discharge on vaginal mucosa and labia

Differential Diagnosis VVC; consider trichomoniasis, BV, MPC

Laboratory Vaginal fluid pH 4.0; amine odor test negative; microscopy of vaginal fluid mixed with KOH solution showed yeasts and pseudohyphae; saline microscopy negative for motile trichomonads; cervical NAATs for *C. trachomatis* and *N. gonorrhoeae* (negative)

Diagnosis VVC

Treatment Fluconazole 150 mg PO (single dose)

Sex Partner Management Patient advised that partner need not be examined unless symptomatic (e.g., penile irritation or rash)

Comment Screening test for *C. trachomatis* was obtained on the basis of age ≤20 years; tests for other STDs optional

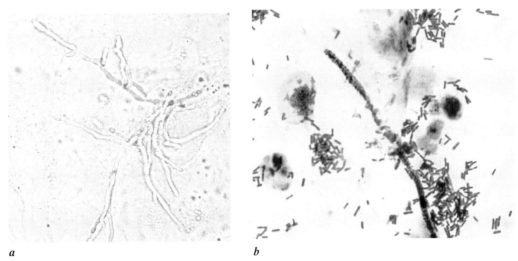

a   *b*

19–2. Microscopic findings in vulvovaginal candidiasis. *a.* 10% KOH digest of vaginal secretions showing pseudo-hyphae of *C. albicans*. (*Courtesy of David A. Eschenbach, M.D.*) *b.* Gram-stained smear of vaginal secretions, showing typically mottled, gram-positive pseudohypha of *C. albicans* and multiple *Lactobacillus* morphotypes. (*Courtesy of Sharon L. Hillier, Ph.D.*). Gram stain and KOH microscopy are similarly effective in diagnosis of VVC.

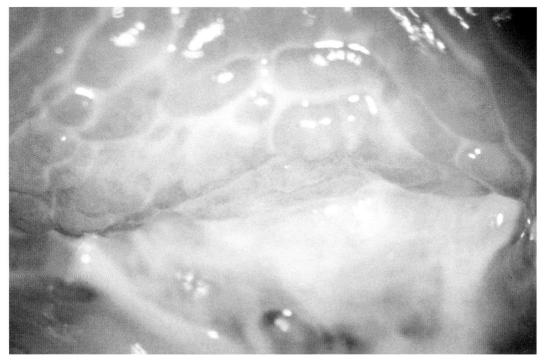

19–3. Bacterial vaginosis; white, homogeneous discharge smoothly coating the vaginal mucosa. (Also see Fig. 10–2.) (*Courtesy of Claire E. Stevens.*)

CASE

Patient Profile Age 22, single, photographer's assistant

History Increased vaginal discharge with unpleasant odor for 1 week; "strong" odor after unprotected vaginal sex; monogamous 1 month with a male partner; history of chlamydia and genital warts 2 years earlier

Examination External genitals normal; homogeneous white vaginal secretions at introitus and smoothly coating vaginal mucosa; cervix showed small area of ectopy, with slightly cloudy mucus in os; bimanual examination normal

Differential Diagnosis Probable BV; consider trichomoniasis, VVC, chlamydia, gonorrhea, physiologic discharge

Laboratory Vaginal fluid pH 5.0; amine (fishy) odor with addition of 10% KOH; saline wet-mount microscopy showed clue cells, no trichomonads, rare PMNs; cervical NAATs for *C. trachomatis* and *N. gonorrhoeae*, RPR, HIV serology (all negative)

Diagnosis Bacterial vaginosis

Treatment Metronidazole 500 mg PO *bid* for 7 days

Partner Management Advised to refer her partner for STD evaluation to exclude other STDs; his examination was normal, not treated

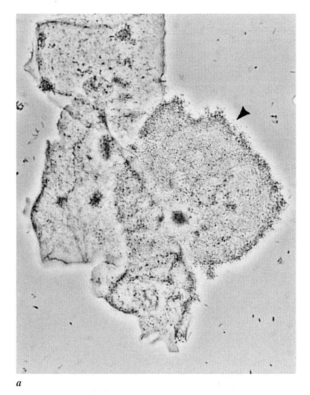

a

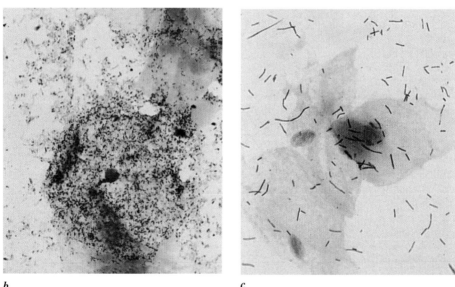

b   *c*

19–4. Microscopic findings in bacterial vaginosis. *a.* Clue cell (arrow) adjacent to normal vaginal epithelial cells. The clue cell has an indistinct, ragged margin and a refractile, granular appearance due to large numbers of adherent bacteria. *b.* Gram-stained smear of secretions in bacterial vaginosis, showing myriads of small, pleomorphic, gram-negative and gram-positive bacteria that heavily coat a clue cell; *Lactobacillus* morphotypes are not seen. *c.* Gram-stained smear of normal vaginal fluid, showing epithelial cells and predominant flora of large, gram-positive bacilli (*Lactobacillus* species). (*Courtesy of David A. Eschenbach, M.D. [a] and Sharon L. Hillier, Ph.D. [b,c].*)

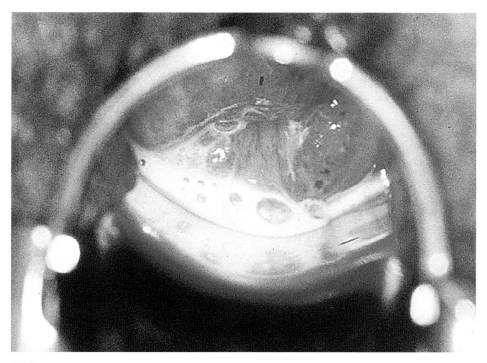

19–5. Purulent vaginal discharge in trichomonal vaginitis. Bubbles due to gas production are seen in a minority of cases but are highly specific for trichomoniasis. Mucopurulent cervical discharge and a small area of edematous cervical ectopy also are present.

CASE

Patient Profile Age 24, single, unemployed, recovering heroin addict, referred from a drug rehabilitation agency

History Increased vaginal discharge and slight vulvar pruritus for 2 weeks; one male partner for 6 months

Examination External genitals normal; copious, malodorous, faintly yellow vaginal discharge with bubbles; small area of cervical ectopy and mucopurulent cervical discharge; no adnexal tenderness or masses

Differential Diagnosis Trichomoniasis, bacterial vaginosis; probable MPC; rule out vulvovaginal candidiasis, gonorrhea, chlamydial infection

Laboratory Vaginal fluid pH 5.5; amine odor test positive; saline preparation showed PMNs, motile trichomonads, few clue cells; Gram-stained endocervical smear showed many PMNs without GND; cultures for *C. trachomatis* (negative) and *N. gonorrhoeae* (positive); VDRL (negative); HIV serology (positive)

Diagnosis Trichomonal vaginitis; gonorrhea with MPC; HIV infection

Treatment Metronidazole 2.0 g PO (single dose); patient was contacted after *N. gonorrhoeae* culture result was reported positive and given cefixime 400 mg PO and azithromycin 1.0 g PO (both single dose)

Partner Management Partner contacted; treated with metronidazole, cefixime, and azithromycin; also found to have gonorrhea, HIV-positive

Comment Trichomoniasis often is associated with other STDs, such as gonorrhea. The clinically evident MPC could be the result of gonorrhea, trichomoniasis, or both. The patient and her partner were referred to an infectious diseases clinic for HIV/AIDS clinical care.

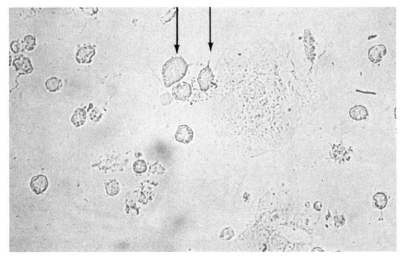

19–6. Saline wet mount microscopy of vaginal secretions in trichomoniasis, showing *T. vaginalis* (arrows) and leukocytes. In actual use, trichomonads are readily distinguished from leukocytes by their motility.

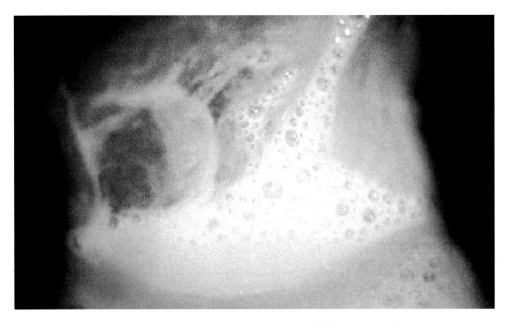

19–7. Frothy vaginal discharge in trichomonal vaginitis. (*Courtesy of Claire E. Stevens.*)

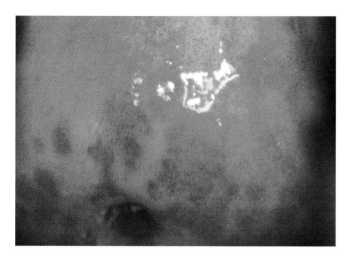

19–8. Cervical petechiae ("colpitis macularis," "strawberry cervix"), an uncommon but specific manifestation of trichomoniasis. (*Reprinted with permission from Holmes KK, et al., eds. Sexually Transmitted Diseases. 3rd ed. New York, NY: McGraw-Hill; 1999.*)

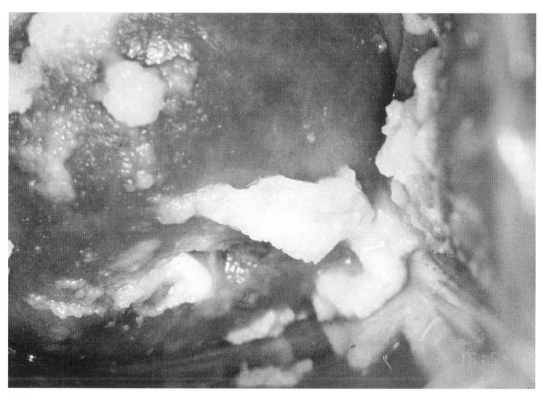

19–9. Clumped vaginal exudate and mucosal erythema in vulvovaginal candidiasis. (*Courtesy of Claire E. Stevens.*)

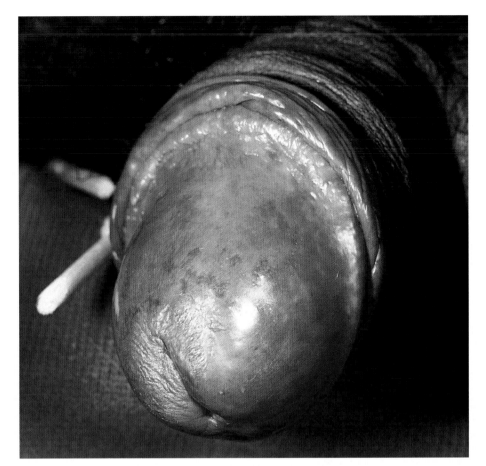

19–10. Balanitis due to *C. albicans* in the uncircumcised partner of a woman with VVC, showing punctate erythema of glans penis.

SUGGESTED READING

Atashili J, et al. Bacterial vaginosis and HIV acquisition: a meta-analysis of published studies. *AIDS.* 2008;22:1493-501. *Documentation of the strong association between BV and incident sexually acquired HIV infection.*

Hillier S, et al. Bacterial vaginosis. Chapter 42 in KK Holmes, et al., eds. *Sexually Transmitted Diseases.* 4th ed. New York, NY: McGraw-Hill; 2008:735-68. *A comprehensive overview of pathogenesis, epidemiology, and clinical manifestations of BV.*

Hobbs MM, et al. *Trichomonas vaginalis* and trichomoniasis. Chapter 43 in KK Holmes, et al., eds. *Sexually Transmitted Diseases.* 4th ed. New York, NY: McGraw-Hill; 2008:771-93. *A comprehensive overview of pathogenesis, epidemiology, and clinical manifestations.*

Holmes KK, et al. Lower genital tract infection syndromes in women. Chapter 55 in KK Holmes, et al., eds. *Sexually Transmitted Diseases.* 4th ed. New York, NY: McGraw-Hill; 2008:987-1016. *A comprehensive, extensively referenced review of cervical, urethral, and vaginal infections in women.*

Johnson VJ, Mabey DC. Global epidemiology and control of *Trichomonas vaginalis. Curr Opin Infect Dis.* 2008;21:56-64. *A comprehensive review of the epidemiology, health impact, and potential value of public health prevention strategies to combat trichomoniasis.*

Schwebke JR. Bacterial vaginosis: are we coming full circle? [Editorial]. *J Infect Dis.* 2009;200:1633-5. *Review of the controversies about the sexually transmitted nature of the syndrome, in accompaniment to a study in the same issue documenting absence of BV in women with neither coital nor noncoital vaginal sexual experience (Fethers KA, et al. J Infect Dis. 2009;200:1662-70).*

Sobel JD. Vulvovaginal candidiasis. Chapter 45 in KK Holmes, et al., eds. *Sexually Transmitted Diseases.* 4th ed. New York, NY: McGraw-Hill; 2008:823-38. *A comprehensive overview of pathogenesis, epidemiology, and clinical manifestations of BV.*

Wendel KA, Workowski KA. Trichomoniasis: challenges to appropriate management. *Clin Infect Dis.* 2007;44(Suppl 3):S123-9. *Review of data in support of CDC's 2006 treatment guidelines.*

Wilson JF. In the clinic: vaginitis and cervicitis. *Ann Intern Med.* 2009;151:ITIC3 1-15. *A comprehensive, well-referenced review of clinical aspects, with a combined syndromic and etiologic approach.*

20

Pelvic Inflammatory Disease

Pelvic inflammatory disease (PID) is the most common serious STD complication, apart from AIDS. PID is defined as salpingitis, usually accompanied by endometritis and sometimes pelvic peritonitis, that results from ascending genital infection unrelated to childbirth or invasive procedures of the genital tract. At least 90% of first episodes of PID meeting these criteria are sexually acquired, but a few cases are attributed to nonsexually transmitted pathogens. The frequency of symptomatic PID appears to have declined in the United States and the United Kingdom since the 1990s, perhaps due in part to expanded chlamydia screening.

The main sequelae of PID are infertility and ectopic pregnancy that result from tubal scarring, and chronic pelvic pain. The risk of infertility following symptomatic PID was estimated in the 1980s to be 15–20%, but this varies with the causative agent, the severity of PID as documented by laparoscopy, and the number of PID episodes. More recent estimates suggest a lower risk of infertility, perhaps the result of earlier diagnosis and improved recognition of mild cases. Each occurrence of PID enhances the risk of subsequent episodes, probably because scarring impairs normal tubal clearance mechanisms. PID is sometimes clinically severe, accompanied by fever, tubo-ovarian abscess, peritonitis, and other systemic manifestations, but most cases are mild. Indeed, subclinical salpingitis is estimated to account for 60% of all cases, and most women with tubal factor infertility or ectopic pregnancy have no past history of PID or unexplained abdominal pain. "Chronic" PID is an indistinct entity; the term sometimes is used inappropriately for pelvic adhesions and unexplained pelvic pain, without evidence of active infection or inflammation.

Chlamydia trachomatis is the most common cause of acute PID in industrialized countries and the likely etiology of most subclinical cases. *Neisseria gonorrhoeae* remains a major cause in populations and geographic settings where gonorrhea is common. *Mycoplasma genitalium* may have an etiologic role in 10–20% of cases, but conflicting results have been reported and its contribution to PID is uncertain, although caution dictates coverage for *M. genitalium* in treatment. Numerous other bacteria contribute to PID, including *M. hominis* and various aerobic and anaerobic components of the vaginal flora, and most women with acute PID have bacterial vaginosis (BV). It is probable that any of several cervical infections—gonorrhea, chlamydial infection, perhaps *M. genitalium*, and perhaps cervicitis associated with BV—result in ascending endometrial and tubal infection with the primary pathogen, vaginal bacteria, or both. No sexually transmitted pathogen can be isolated in most cases of recurrent PID. Occasionally a nonsexually transmitted pathogen such as *Haemophilus influenzae* is isolated in pure culture from the fallopian tubes or culdocentesis aspirate in women with primary PID. The specific bacteria contributing to salpingitis usually are not known in individual patients, and antibiotic treatment should cover *C. trachomatis*, *N. gonorrhoeae*, *M. genitalium*, and mixed aerobic and anaerobic flora.

EPIDEMIOLOGY

Incidence and Prevalence

- Diagnosed in 1–5% of women in STD clinics in the United States
- Declining rates in the United States and United Kingdom since 1990s
  - In the United Kingdom, the rate of PID in general practices declined 10% per year from 2000 to 2008, especially in women age 16-19 years.
  - In the United States, estimated annual rate declined 25% in women with private health insurance, from 317 cases per 100,000 in 2001 to 336 per 100,000 in 2005
  - Perhaps due in part to improved prevention of chlamydial infections and gonorrhea; probably also influenced by changing definitions and diagnostic standards
- Overt or subclinical PID is the most common cause of ectopic pregnancy and tubal infertility

Transmission

- As for *C. trachomatis* and *N. gonorrhoeae* (see Chaps. 3 and 4)
- Uncommon in sexually inactive women, but nonsexually acquired cases occur, especially in recurrent PID

Age

- Markedly elevated risk in sexually active teens, probably due to both behavioral and physiologic factors that may enhance susceptibility to *C. trachomatis* and perhaps *N. gonorrhoeae* (e.g., cervical ectopy)

Sexual Orientation

- Probably uncommon in WSW with exclusively female sex partners, but few data exist

Other Risk Factors

- Behavioral markers of STD risk
- Some intrauterine contraceptive devices (especially older designs) probably increase risk
- Previous PID
- Vaginal douching
- Repeat chlamydial infection may elevate PID risk compared to initial infection

HISTORY

Incubation Period

- Varies from 1–2 days to several months following acquisition of *C. trachomatis* or *N. gonorrhoeae*

Symptoms

- Most cases mild or subclinical
- Low abdominal pain is nearly universal in symptomatic cases
- Most patients have increased vaginal discharge or other symptoms of MPC or BV (see Chaps. 18 and 19)
- Often dyspareunia, menorrhagia, intermenstrual bleeding
- Right upper quadrant abdominal pain (Fitz-Hugh–Curtis syndrome)
- Fever, chills, malaise, nausea, and vomiting in severe cases

PHYSICAL EXAMINATION

- Pelvic adnexal tenderness, usually bilateral; variable severity
- Uterine fundal and cervical motion tenderness
- Signs of MPC or BV
- Fever is common but often absent
- Lower quadrant abdominal tenderness, sometimes with rebound tenderness or other peritoneal inflammatory signs; usually bilateral
- Adnexal mass sometimes present on bimanual examination
- Right upper quadrant tenderness may be elicited, due to perihepatitis (Fitz-Hugh-Curtis syndrome), especially with chlamydial PID

LABORATORY DIAGNOSIS

Lower Genital Tract Infection and Microbiology

- Laboratory evidence of MPC, BV, or both usually is present (see Chaps. 18 and 19)
- NAAT or culture for *N. gonorrhoeae* and *C. trachomatis*
- If laparoscopy done, test tubal aspirate or peritoneal exudate for *N. gonorrhoeae* and *C. trachomatis* and culture for aerobic and anaerobic bacteria

Other Tests

- Leukocyte count and either erythrocyte sedimentation rate (ESR) or assay for C-reactive protein (CRP) should be performed; normal results do not exclude PID, but elevated levels are associated with increased severity
- Pelvic ultrasound examination
- Laparoscopy indicated if diagnosis is uncertain, in severe cases, or when initial response to antibiotics is inadequate
- Endometrial biopsy can be helpful in documenting endometritis, a surrogate marker of salpingitis

DIAGNOSTIC CRITERIA

- In sexually active women, low abdominal pain plus adnexal or cervical motion tenderness indicate sufficient likelihood of PID to warrant presumptive treatment
- Ancillary criteria enhance specificity of the diagnosis
  - Fever (≥101°F or 38.0°C)
  - Mucopurulent cervicitis
  - Purulent vaginal discharge
  - Abundant PMNs in cervical or vaginal discharge
  - Elevated ESR or CRP
  - Cervical infection with *C. trachomatis* or *N. gonorrhoeae*
- Laparoscopy may be helpful, but only ~70% of patients with clinically diagnosed PID have laparoscopic evidence of salpingitis

TREATMENT

Principles

- Treat all suspected cases while awaiting diagnostic confirmation
- Routinely cover *N. gonorrhoeae*, *C. trachomatis*, and mixed aerobic and anaerobic bacteria, regardless of pathogens identified in patient or sex partner and regardless of apparent clinical severity
- All recommended antibiotic regimens have similar short-term clinical efficacy
- No comparative data are available on long-term outcomes, i.e., prevention of infertility, ectopic pregnancy, or recurrent PID
- Indications for hospitalization and parenteral therapy
  - Inability to reliably exclude surgical emergency (e.g., appendicitis)
  - Suspected tubo-ovarian abscess
  - Pregnancy
  - Severe clinical manifestations such as nausea, vomiting, high fever, or peritonitis
  - Low likelihood of adherence to oral antibiotic therapy
  - Poor clinical response to initial oral antibiotics

Recommended Regimens

Inpatient Treatment

For patients with PID of sufficient severity to require hospitalization, many experts recommend Regimen A for probable chlamydial or gonococcal PID and Regimen B when predominant aerobic and anaerobic infection is likely (e.g., recurrent PID or suspected tubo-ovarian abscess).

- Regimen A
  - Doxycycline 100 mg IV or PO* every 12 hours

---

*Doxycycline administered IV or PO provides similar blood levels; oral therapy may be used if tolerated.

plus

- ○ Cefotetan 2.0 g IV every 12 hours OR cefoxitin 2.0 g IV every 6 hours for minimum 48 hours, or longer until clinical improvement observed

followed by

- ○ Doxycycline 100 mg PO *bid* to complete 14 days total therapy

- Regimen B

  - ○ Clindamycin 900 mg IV every 8 hours for minimum 48 hours or until improved

plus

- ○ Gentamicin 2.0 mg/kg body weight (loading dose) IV or IM, then 1.5 mg/kg IV or IM every 8 hours for a minimum of 48 hours, until improved

followed by

- ○ Doxycycline 100 mg PO *bid* to complete 14 days total therapy; *or*
- ○ Clindamycin 450 mg PO *qid* to complete 14 days total therapy; *or*
- ○ Both doxycycline and clindamycin to complete 14 days total therapy

- Alternative parenteral regimens, providing coverage for all likely pathogens but less well studied

  - ○ Ampicillin/sulbactam 3 g IV every 6 hours plus doxycycline 100 mg IV or PO every 12 hours for ≥48 hours, then oral doxycycline to complete 14 days total therapy

or

- ○ Azithromycin 500 mg IV, followed by azithromycin 250 mg PO once daily for 5–6 days, optionally combined with metronidazole 500 mg PO *bid* for 14 days

Outpatient Treatment

- Initial single dose cephalosporin

  - ○ Ceftriaxone 250 mg IM (single dose)

or

- ○ Cefoxitin 2.0 g IM or IV (single dose) with probenecid 1.0 g PO (single dose)

plus

- ○ Doxycycline 100 mg PO *bid* for 14 days
- ○ Optionally add metronidazole 500 mg PO *bid* for 14 days

Supportive Therapy

- If IUD present, consider removal
- Bed rest may speed subjective improvement in severe cases
- Analgesics as needed
- Advise sexual abstention for at least 2 weeks

Follow-up

- Reexamine every 1–3 days until improved
- Clinical progression at any time or failure to improve within 3–4 days is an indication for laparoscopic diagnosis and parenteral therapy
- After improvement begins, reexamine weekly until clinically resolved

Partner Management

- Examine all partners, even when sexual acquisition of PID seems unlikely
- Treat partners for presumptive gonorrhea and chlamydial infection, unless sexual acquisition is excluded with certainty

Counseling

- Counsel patient about sexually transmitted nature of PID and risks of tubal infertility and ectopic pregnancy
  - Avoid nonspecific terms that deemphasize the sexually transmitted nature of PID (e.g., "infected ovarian cyst")

PARTNER MANAGEMENT AND PREVENTION

- Depending on suspected or documented cause, manage partners as described for gonorrhea, chlamydial infection, or NGU (See Chaps. 3, 4, and 15)
- General STD prevention measures (partner selection, condoms)
- Screen sexually active young women for *C. trachomatis* and *N. gonorrhoeae* (See Chaps. 3 and 4)

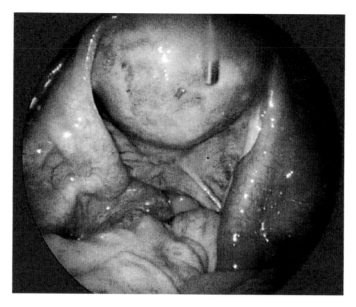

20–1. Laparoscopic view of pelvic structures in acute PID, showing normal uterus being retracted anteriorly by probe; left fallopian tube (left side of figure) has slight edema with reddened, agglutinated fimbria; right tube is moderately swollen; erythematous; purulent exudate is seen deep in cul-de-sac. (*Courtesy of David E. Soper, M.D.*)

CASE

Patient Profile Age 18, grocery clerk

History Increased vaginal discharge for 10 days; mild low abdominal pain for 4 days, exacerbated during intercourse; severe pain for 1 day; no fever or chills; monogamous with current boyfriend for 3 months

Examination Afebrile; bilateral lower quadrant abdominal tenderness, without rebound; external genitals normal; edematous cervical ectopy and mucopurulent cervical exudate; homogeneous white vaginal fluid; moderate cervical motion, fundal and adnexal tenderness bilaterally; left adnexal fullness without overt mass

Differential Diagnosis Pelvic inflammatory disease, ectopic pregnancy, endometriosis, appendicitis, urinary tract infection (UTI), colitis

Laboratory Findings of BV and MPC by microscopy, pH, and amine odor test (see Chaps 18 and 19); WBC 8,600 per mm^3 with normal differential; ESR 35 mm/h; endocervical NAATs for *C. trachomatis* (positive) and *N. gonorrhoeae* (negative); RPR and HIV serology negative

Diagnosis PID due to *C. trachomatis*

Treatment Ceftriaxone 250 mg IM (single dose), followed by doxycycline 100 mg PO *bid* and metronidazole 500 mg PO *bid* for 14 days

Partner Management Advised to refer partner for examination and treatment; he was found to have asymptomatic urethral chlamydial infection; treated with azithromycin 1.0 g PO, single dose

Follow-up Reexamined 2 days later; pain improved, with reduced abdominal and adnexal tenderness; counseled regarding STD prevention and future risks of infertility and ectopic pregnancy; scheduled to be rescreened for *C. trachomatis* 3 months later.

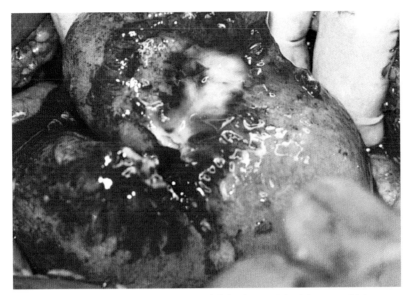

20–2. Tubo-ovarian abscess in severe PID: bilobed pyosalpinx/abscess, which was adherent to uterine fundus (above center), purulent exudate at the site where the uterus and pyosalpinx adhered. (*Courtesy of David E. Soper, M.D., reprinted with permission from* Am J Obstet Gynecol *1991;164:1370-6.*)

CASE

Patient Profile Age 32, married schoolteacher

History Intermittent, mild low abdominal pain and vaginal discharge since IUD inserted 4 months earlier; severe abdominal pain, fever, chills, nausea, and vomiting for 1 day; denied extramarital sex partners

Examination Temperature 39.2°C; bilateral lower quadrant direct and rebound abdominal tenderness; profuse mucopurulent cervical discharge; IUD string observed; marked bilateral pelvic tenderness, with suggestion of right adnexal mass (examination compromised by tenderness and guarding)

Differential Diagnosis PID, appendicitis, ectopic pregnancy, severe endometriosis

Laboratory Pelvic ultrasound showed 6 × 8-cm fluid-filled mass with internal echoes, plus small effusion in cul-de-sac; WBC 14,700 per mm³ with 80% PMNs; ESR 50 mm/h; Gram-stained smear of cervical exudate and vaginal saline mount showed many PMNs and clue cells, without trichomonads or yeasts; vaginal pH 5.0, KOH amine odor positive; negative cultures for *N. gonorrhoeae* and *C. trachomatis*; 2 blood cultures sent (negative); VDRL and HIV serology negative

Diagnosis Acute PID with tubo-ovarian abscess, following IUD insertion; bacterial vaginosis

Treatment Patient hospitalized; IUD removed; treated with clindamycin and gentamicin IV for 4 days until improvement began, then clindamycin 450 mg PO *qid* to complete 14 days treatment

Partner Management Husband referred for examination; denied other sex partners, examination normal; negative urine NAATs for *C. trachomatis* and *N. gonorrhoeae* (negative); not treated

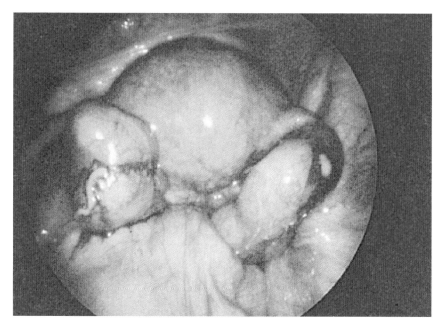

20–3. Bilateral pyosalpinx in severe PID; pus is seen exuding from both tubes at sites of needle aspiration for culture. (*Courtesy of David E. Soper, M.D.; reprinted with permission from* Am J Obstet Gynecol *1991;164:1370-6.*)

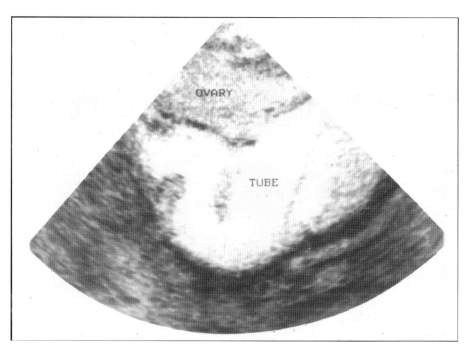

20–4. Pelvic ultrasound examination in acute PID with pyosalpinx. (*Courtesy of Faye Laing, M.D.*)

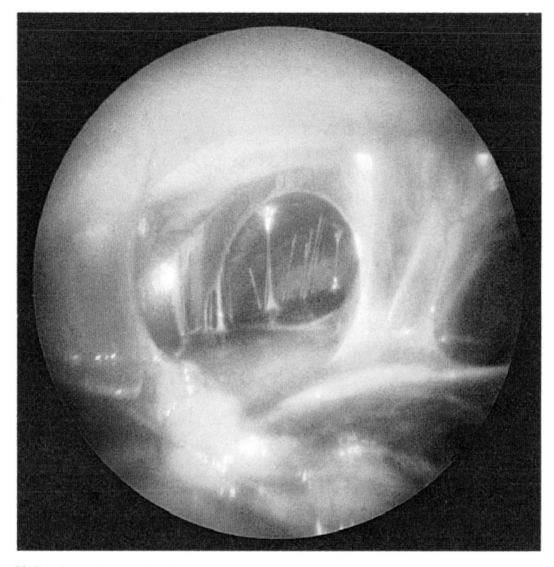

20–5. Adhesions between liver (below) and parietal peritoneum in a woman with acute perihepatitis (Fitz-Hugh–Curtis syndrome) due to *C. trachomatis*. (*Courtesy of David E. Soper, M.D.*)

SUGGESTED READING

French CE, et al. Estimation of the rate of pelvic inflammatory disease: trends in England, 2000-2008. *Sex Transm Dis.* 2011;38:158-62. *A well done analysis of the UK General Practice Research Database.*

Haggarty CL, et al. Risk of sequelae after *Chlamydia trachomatis* genital infection in women. *J Infect Dis.* 2010;201(Suppl 2):S134-55. *A comprehensive literature review on chlamydial PID and its main consequences, infertility and ectopic pregnancy.*

Judlin P. Current concepts in managing pelvic inflammatory disease. *Curr Opin Infect Dis.* 2010;23: 83-7. *An up-to-date review of the literature on PID treatment.*

Oakeshott P, et al. Randomised controlled trial of screening for *Chlamydia trachomatis* to prevent pelvic inflammatory disease: the POPI (prevention of pelvic infection) trial. *BMJ.* 2010;340:c1642. *A study showing benefit of chlamydia screening in PID prevention (controversially interpreted by the authors as showing marginal benefit); a useful introduction to public health chlamydia prevention strategies.*

Paavonen J, et al. Pelvic inflammatory disease. Chapter 57 in KK Holmes, et al., eds. *Sexually Transmitted Diseases.* 4th ed. New York, NY: McGraw-Hill; 2008:1017-50. *A comprehensive review in the premier textbook on STD.*

Scholes D, et al. Prevention of pelvic inflammatory disease by screening for cervical chlamydial infection. *N Engl J Med.* 1996;334:1362-6. *A prospective study documenting reduced incidence of symptomatic PID in women screened for chlamydial infection; a central underpinning of chlamydia prevention strategies.*

21

Proctitis, Colitis, and Enteritis

Sexually acquired proctitis can be caused by *Neisseria gonorrhoeae, Chlamydia trachomatis*, herpes simplex virus (HSV), and *Treponema pallidum*. Most such infections are acquired by direct exposure through anal intercourse, but some cases in women probably result from anal exposure to infected cervicovaginal secretions, and some infections among men who have sex with men (MSM) may be transmitted by direct exchange of anorectal secretions by fingers or sex toys. Enteritis, or small intestinal infection, can be sexually acquired by practices that foster oral exposure to feces. Giardiasis, salmonellosis, cryptosporidiosis, microsporidiosis, isosporiasis, and norovirus gastroenteritis are examples of sexually transmissible enteric infections. Colitis and proctocolitis are acquired sexually either from fecal–oral contamination, e.g., amebiasis and shigellosis, or by rectal inoculation, e.g., lymphogranuloma venereum (LGV). *Campylobacter* infection and salmonellosis, acquired orally, may result in enteritis, colitis, or both syndromes (enterocolitis). All sexually active persons are susceptible to these infections, but the practices conducive to their transmission are most frequent among MSM, who comprise the majority of patients with these syndromes. Sexually transmitted enteritis, colitis, and proctocolitis are clinically indistinguishable from similar syndromes acquired nonsexually, such as inflammatory bowel disease and numerous foodborne or waterborne infections. In patients with AIDS, colitis is often caused by cytomegalovirus (CMV) and other opportunistic pathogens.

EPIDEMIOLOGY

Incidence and Prevalence

- Highly variable, depending on sexual practices
- Reliable statistics not available

Transmission

- Receptive anal intercourse
- Sexual practices that risk fecal–oral contamination (e.g., analingus, contaminated hands, or sex toys)

- Rectal STDs in women probably can be acquired via anal contamination with infected cervicovaginal secretions
- LGV among MSM apparently has been transmitted by direct rectal contamination through hands and sex toys; the same mechanism probably explains some other rectal STDs in MSM

Age

- No specific predilection

Sex and Sexual Orientation

- Sexually transmitted gastrointestinal STDs are most common in MSM

HISTORY

Incubation Period

- Variable, depending on specific infection

Symptoms
Proctitis

- Anorectal pain, tenesmus, constipation, bleeding
- Mucus or purulent exudate may be observed during defecation or on feces
- Anal or perianal vesiculopustular lesions or ulcers (suggest herpes or syphilis)
- Fever or systemic symptoms (suggest primary herpes or LGV)
- Sacral neuropathy (e.g., bladder paralysis; suggests primary herpes)

Colitis

- Diarrhea, sometimes bloody
- Abdominal cramps
- Often fever or other systemic symptoms

Enteritis

- Diarrhea, usually without cramping
- Variable degrees of nausea, vomiting, anorexia, bloating, flatulence, weight loss, fever

Proctocolitis and Enterocolitis

- Simultaneous symptoms of the component syndromes

Epidemiologic History

- History of exposure
- Sexual practices that foster anorectal or fecal–oral exposure

PHYSICAL EXAMINATION

Proctitis

- Anoscopy or sigmoidoscopy showing mucosal erythema, extending ≤10 cm above anus
- Purulent exudate, typically observed in anal crypts
- Mucosal ulcers or petechiae

- Bleeding induced by swabbing rectal mucosa ("wipe test")
- Ulcers or vesiculopustules of anal canal or perianally

Colitis and Proctocolitis

- Abdominal tenderness, usually maximal in left lower quadrant
- Sigmoidoscopy or colonoscopy typically demonstrates inflammation >10 cm above the anus
- Proctocolitis causes clinical signs and mucosal changes consistent with both proctitis and colitis
- Fever is common

Enteritis and Enterocolitis

- Often no physical findings
- Sometimes abdominal tenderness or enhanced bowel sounds

DIFFERENTIAL AND LABORATORY DIAGNOSIS

Proctitis

- Most MSM with acute proctitis have gonorrhea, chlamydial infection (including LGV), herpes, or primary or secondary syphilis
- Differential diagnosis probably is similar in sexually active women, but poorly studied
- Anoscopy for visual inspection and clinical specimens
  - Gram-stained smear of rectal secretions
  - NAAT or cultures for *N. gonorrhoeae*
  - NAAT or culture for *C. trachomatis*
  - NAAT or culture for HSV
  - Serological test for syphilis
  - Type-specific HSV serology
  - Darkfield examination if ulcers or other lesions consistent with syphilis observed
  - Rectal biopsy if diagnosis remains obscure

Colitis and Proctocolitis

- Usual causes are *C. trachomatis* (especially LGV strains), *Campylobacter jejuni*, *Shigella* species, *Salmonella* species, and *Entamoeba histolytica*
- Clinically indistinguishable from ulcerative colitis or Crohn disease
  - Perform sigmoidoscopy or colonoscopy
  - NAAT or culture for *N. gonorrhoeae*
  - NAAT or culture for *C. trachomatis*
  - NAAT or culture for HSV
- Examine stool for leukocytes, culture for enteric pathogens, and ova and parasite examination
- Chlamydia/LGV serology
- Biopsy if diagnosis remains obscure; LGV may be histologically indistinguishable from Crohn disease

Enteritis and Enterocolitis

- Broad differential diagnosis
  - Among MSM, *Giardia lamblia* probably is most common cause of enteritis without colitis
  - *Campylobacter*
  - *Salmonella*
  - *Cryptosporidium, Isospora, Cyclospora*, microsporidia, CMV, and *Mycobacterium avium* complex are potential etiologies in HIV-infected and other immunocompromised persons
- Examine stool for leukocytes
- Stool culture for enteric pathogens
- Ova and parasite examination
- Consider "string test" of duodenal secretions for *G. lamblia*
- Colonoscopy, upper gastrointestinal endoscopy, and mucosal biopsy often are indicated

TREATMENT

Proctitis and Proctocolitis

- Treat according to specific etiology
- Depending on clinical severity and available epidemiologic information, presumptive therapy may be indicated while awaiting diagnostic test results:
  - Ulcerative proctitis that suggests syphilis or herpes: Benzathine penicillin plus valacyclovir or acyclovir: (see Chaps. 5 and 8)
  - Proctitis or proctocolitis without mucocutaneous ulceration: Ceftriaxone plus doxycycline for presumptive chlamydia or gonorrhea (see Chaps. 3 and 4)
  - Suspected LGV: Doxycycline 100 mg PO *bid* for 3 weeks (see Chap. 3)

Colitis and Enterocolitis
Amebiasis

- Overt colitis or other suspicion of invasive amebiasis
  - Metronidazole 750 mg PO *tid* for 10 days
  followed by
  - Iodoquinol 650 mg PO *tid* for 3 weeks
- Asymptomatic carriage
  - Iodoquinol 650 mg PO *tid* for 3 weeks
  or
  - Paromomycin 10 mg/kg body weight *tid* plus diloxanide furoate 500 mg PO *tid* for 3 weeks

Salmonellosis

- Most cases resolve without antimicrobial therapy
- If indicated by severe infection, pending susceptibility test results:
  - Ciprofloxacin 500 mg PO *bid* for 7 days, *or*
  - Other fluoroquinolone regimen in equivalent dosage

Shigellosis

- Most cases resolve without antimicrobial therapy
- If indicated by severe infection, pending susceptibility test results:
  - Ciprofloxacin 500 mg PO *bid* for 7 days, *or*
  - Other fluoroquinolone regimen in equivalent dosage

Campylobacter Infection

- Mild cases usually require no treatment
- Severe infections
  - Azithromycin 500 mg PO once daily for 3 days

  or

  - Erythromycin 500 mg PO *qid* for 7 days

Enteritis
Giardiasis

- Metronidazole 250–500 mg PO *tid* for 7 days

  or

- Paromomycin 500 mg PO *tid* for 7–10 days

  or

- Furazolidone 100 mg PO *qid* for 7–10 days

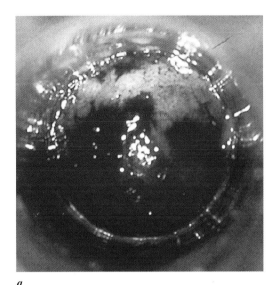
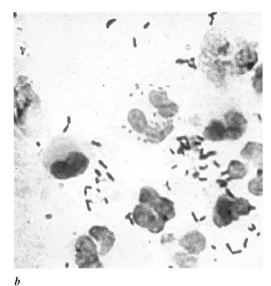

a   *b*

21–1. *a.* Gonococcal proctitis: anoscopic view of purulent exudate and mucosal bleeding (positive "wipe test"). *b.* Gram-stained smear of rectal exudate, showing a single PMN with ICGND. (*Part b reprinted with permission from Holmes KK, et al, eds. Sexually Transmitted Diseases. 3rd ed. New York, NY: McGraw-Hill; 1999.*)

CASE

Patient Profile Age 34, unemployed, methamphetamine-addicted gay man

History Anal itching, discharge, and blood mixed in stool for 3 days; no diarrhea, cramps, fever, or systemic symptoms; frequent unprotected sex with anonymous partners

Examination Genitals normal; anus normal; anoscopy showed purulent exudate and mucosal friability with spontaneous bleeding, enhanced by swabbing (positive "wipe test")

Differential Diagnosis Gonorrhea, herpes, chlamydial infection (including LGV), syphilis

Laboratory Gram stain of rectal exudate showed PMNs, some with ICGND; rectal culture for *N. gonorrhoeae* (positive); rectal cultures for *C. trachomatis* and HSV (both negative); darkfield examination, stat RPR, VDRL, HIV serology (all negative)

Diagnosis Gonococcal proctitis

Treatment Cefixime 400 mg PO, single dose, plus azithromycin 1.0 g PO, single dose

Partner Management Patient was unable to identify sex partners

Comment The patient was seen before resurgent LGV appeared in MSM in the 2000s, and before current recommendations of ceftriaxone for gonorrhea. Today work-up for acute proctitis would include NAAT for *C. trachomatis* and LGV serology, and treatment with ceftriaxone 250 mg IM instead of cefixime (see Chaps. 3 and 4). Although Gram-stained smears of anal secretions are optional, microscopic examination of anoscopically obtained specimens may be useful, especially if purulent exudate is observed and directly sampled. In this patient, the smear permitted presumptive diagnosis and immediate specific therapy for gonorrhea. The patient's symptoms resolved over the next 2 days, but he returned 2 weeks later with sore throat, fever, cervical lymphadenopathy, and a faint generalized maculopapular skin rash; primary HIV infection was diagnosed. Had he presented in 2010, HIV serology would have included NAAT for HIV RNA, perhaps permitting diagnosis of his acute HIV infection at the initial visit (see Chap. 12).

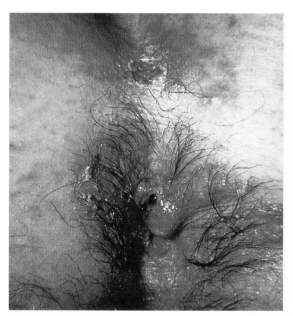

a

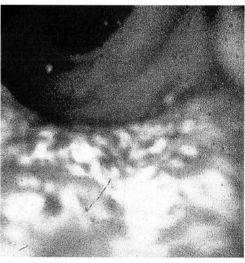

b

21–2. Acute proctitis due to primary herpes in a man who presented 8 days after receptive anal sex with a new partner, with 5 days of increasing perianal pain, tenesmus, difficulty urinating, fever, and headache. *a.* Ulcer of perineum anterior to anus, with anal edema and erythema. *b.* Mucosal ulcers and exudate viewed by fiberoptic sigmoidoscopy. (*Part b courtesy of Christina M. Surawicz, M.D.*) Also see Fig. 8–8.

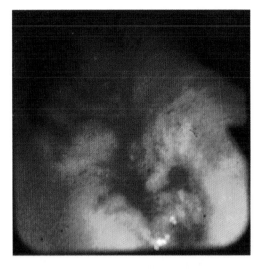

21–3. Proctitis due to *Chlamydia trachomatis* (non–LGV strain), showing mucosal erythema and edema, viewed by fiberoptic sigmoidoscopy. (*Courtesy of Thomas Quinn, M.D.*)

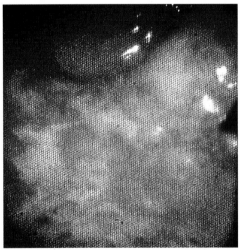

21–4. Gonococcal proctitis: purulent rectal exudate viewed by fiberoptic sigmoidoscopy. (*Courtesy of Christina M. Surawicz, M.D.*)

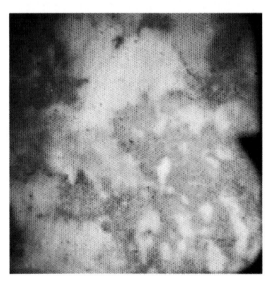

21–5. Amebic proctocolitis: rectal mucosal ulcerations, exudate, and petechiae due to amebic proctocolitis, viewed by fiberoptic sigmoidoscopy. Note similarity to herpetic and gonococcal proctitis (see Figs. 21–2, 21–4). (*Courtesy of Thomas Quinn, M.D.*)

SUGGESTED READING

Felt-Bersma RJ, Bartelsman JF. Haemorrhoids, rectal prolapse, anal fissure, peri-anal fistulae and sexually transmitted diseases. *Best Pract Res Clin Gastroenterol.* 2009;23:575-92. *A comprehensive, clinically oriented, well-illustrated review of anorectal conditions, including those common in MSM and in the differential diagnosis of anorectal STDs.*

Rompalo AM, Quinn TC. Sexually transmitted intestinal syndromes. Chapter 68 in KK Holmes et al, eds. *Sexually Transmitted Diseases.* 4th ed. New York, NY: McGraw-Hill; 2008:1277-1308. *A comprehensive review in the main textbook on sexually transmitted diseases.*

White JA. Manifestations and management of lymphogranuloma venereum. *Curr Opin Infect Dis.* 2009;22:57-66. *A literature review of re-emergent LGV in MSM.*

22

Nonsexually Transmitted Genital Conditions

Many dermatologic conditions can affect the genitals, and some anatomic variants, both genital and nongenital, may be mistaken for abnormal conditions by patients or their health care providers. Not surprisingly, sexually active persons with genital symptoms often present to providers with concerns about STD. Entire textbooks have been written on the topic of genital dermatology, and it is beyond the scope of this book to provide a comprehensive overview. Examples of a few conditions are presented, with emphasis on those that are likely to affect younger persons or are easily confused with STDs.

Fixed Drug Eruption

Fixed drug eruption (FDE) is a localized reaction to a systemic allergen that often involves the genitals. The tetracyclines are among the common causes, and owing to the frequent use of doxycycline and other tetracyclines in STD treatment and the high frequency of genital involvement, tetracycline-related FDEs are common in STD-related clinical practices. Other common causes of FDE include the sulfonamides, metronidazole, phenytoin, and phenolphthalein. The lesion typically resembles a burn, with initial pain and erythema and sometimes bulla formation, followed by superficial sloughing. Repeat FDE may recur in the same location as prior episodes. The reaction usually begins 7–10 days after initiating the offending drug, but with subsequent exposures the onset may be faster, sometimes within hours. Healing occurs without scarring, although hyperpigmentation may persist. Aside from discontinuing the offending drug, no specific treatment is available.

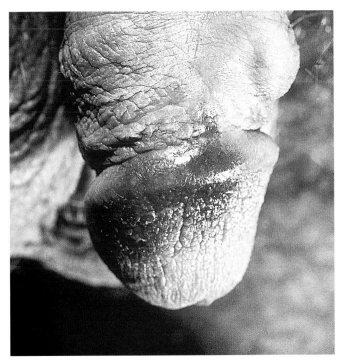

22–1. Fixed drug eruption of the penis. The patient had just finished a 7-day course of tetracycline HCl for NGU and complained of 3 days of pain "like a burn."

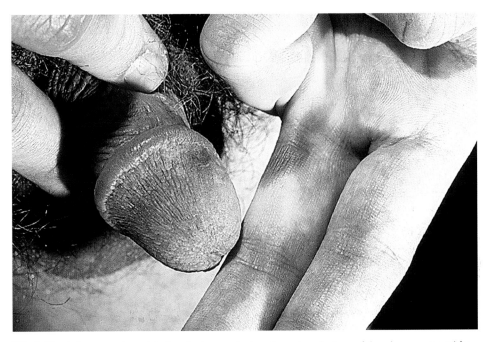

22–2. Fixed drug eruption, with sharply demarcated erythematous lesions of the glans penis and finger web in a patient treated with doxycycline for chlamydial infection.

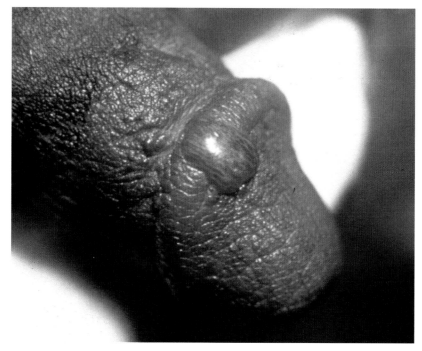

22–3. Fixed drug eruption presenting as a bulla of the glans penis. (*Courtesy of Jeffrey Meffert, M.D.*)

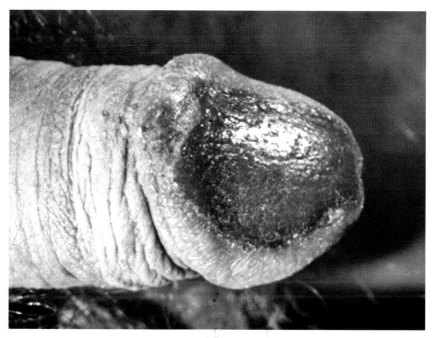

22–4. Fixed drug eruption of the penis.

Psoriasis

Psoriasis often involves the genitals and can mimic secondary syphilis (see Fig. 5–13), scabies (see Fig. 14–2), and keratoderma blennorrhagica of reactive arthritis (see Figs. 17–2 and 17–4). In addition to genital lesions, most patients with psoriasis have lesions of other commonly involved sites, such as the scalp and extensor surfaces of the elbows and knees, or pitted fingernails or toenails. All these areas should be carefully inspected. However, genital lesions may be the first or only manifestation. Sometimes biopsy is necessary for diagnosis.

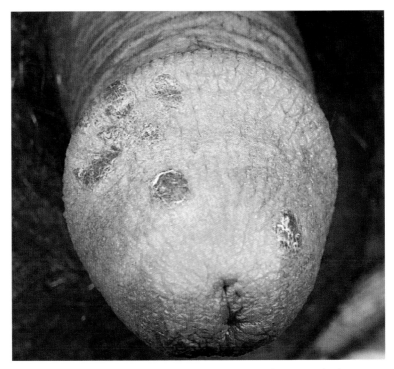

22–5. Psoriasis of the penis. Having begun a new sexual relationship 2 weeks previously, the patient suspected STD; he also had a previously unrecognized patch of typical psoriasis of the scalp.

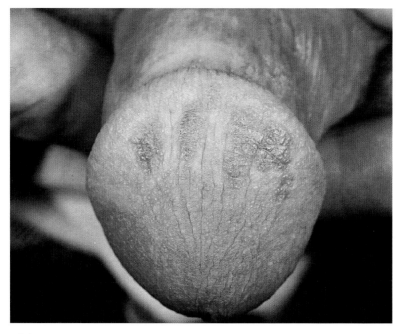

22–6. Psoriasis of the penis.

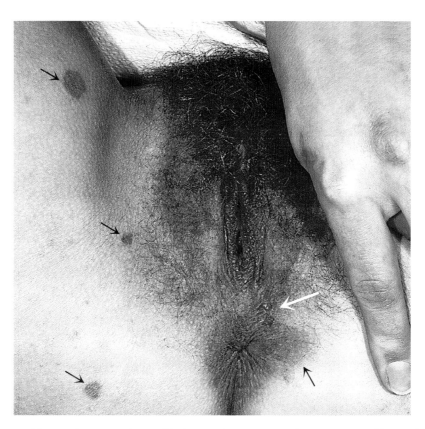

22–7. Psoriasis, with several psoriatic plaques (black arrows) in a woman with recurrent genital herpes (white arrow).

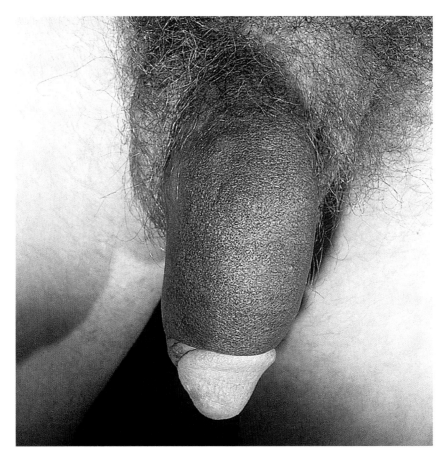

22–8. Penile hemorrhage due to corpus cavernosum fracture. The patient presented to an STD clinic immediately following acute pain and swelling that began after his partner rolled onto his erect penis.

Penile Fracture

Penile fracture is rupture of a corpus cavernosum, a rare event caused by forcible flexion of the penis when erect. Surgery often is required to repair the capsule of the ruptured corpus in order to preserve erection without deformation.

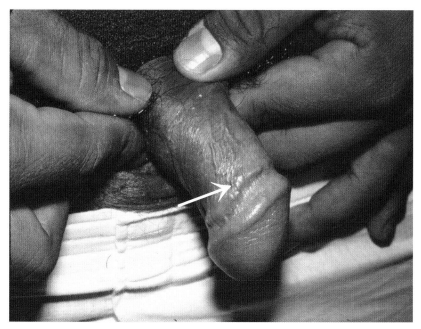

22–9. Sclerosing lymphangitis of the penis (arrow). (*Courtesy of Ted Rosen, M.D. and Journal of the American Academy of Dermatology. 2003;49:916-7; reprinted with permission.*)

Penile Sclerosing Lymphangitis

Sclerosing lymphangitis of the penis sometimes follows vigorous sexual activity and presents as a firm, mobile, painless, elongated, subcutaneous mass typically in the coronal sulcus. Some cases may be slightly painful. No specific treatment is required; the mass typically resolves spontaneously over several weeks. Anecdotal reports suggest the condition is commonly associated with STDs, and up to 25% of patients are said to have gonorrhea, chlamydia, NGU, herpes or other STDs. Although this may be an artifact of STD clinic attendance by young men with genital lesions, it is reasonable to screen young men (age 20–40 years) with the syndrome for common STDs.

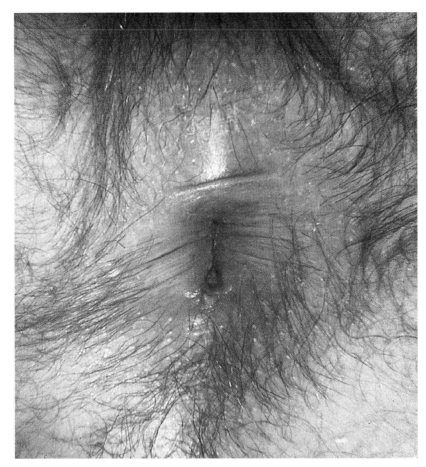

22–10. Anal fissure in a man presenting with anal pain and occasional bleeding for 1 week. (*Courtesy of Steven J. Medwell, M.D.*)

Anal Fissure

Anal fissures are common in all populations and probably are the most frequent cause of ulcerative lesions of the anus. Fissures may be initiated by trauma and probably are particularly frequent in men or women who participate in receptive anal intercourse. Anal fissures may be indistinguishable from syphilitic chancres (see Fig. 5–10) and herpes (see Fig. 8–15). Sexually active persons who present with anal fissures should be asked about receptive anal sex and, if exposed, evaluated for STD.

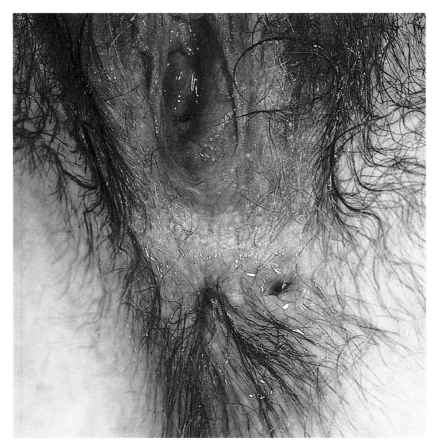

22–11. Chronic rectal fistula with secondary gonococcal infection of the fistula tract.

Perianal Fistula

One year prior to presentation, this woman (Fig. 22-11) had a "boil" near her anus that drained spontaneously. Subsequently, there was a persistent "bump" that periodically drained small amounts of fluid and perhaps feces. She presented to an STD clinic with 1 week of pain and increased drainage from the lesion. A rectal fistula was diagnosed; *Neisseria gonorrhoeae* was isolated from her cervix, anal canal, and the fistula tract.

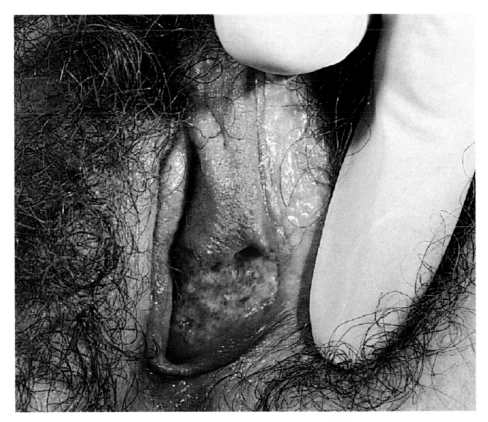

22–12. Genital ulcer due to Behçet syndrome in a 23-year-old woman born in Turkey, who presented to an STD clinic fearing genital herpes. She also reported several years of severe recurrent oral aphthous ulcers.

Behçet Syndrome

Behçet syndrome is a rare condition of probable autoimmune origin, occurring most frequently in persons of Mediterranean ancestry. It is manifested by recurrent oral and genital ulcers which may be deeply erosive, and often by conjunctivitis or uveitis. Complications include arthritis, erythema nodosum, cranial neuropathies, cranial arteritis, meningoencephalitis, stroke, blindness from retinal infarction, and psychosis. Treatment options include colchicine, corticosteroids, chlorambucil, other cytotoxic drugs, and biological antitumor necrosis factor-alpha drugs such as infliximab or etanercept.

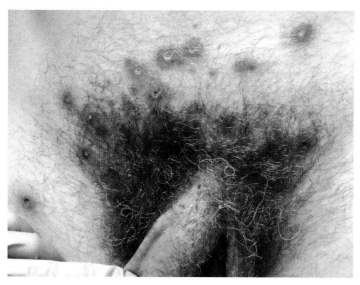

22–13. Methicillin-resistant *Staphylococcus aureus* folliculitis of the pubic area and upper penile shaft. Pustular lesions and ulcers are limited to hair-bearing areas. (*Courtesy of Susan Szabo, PA-C.*)

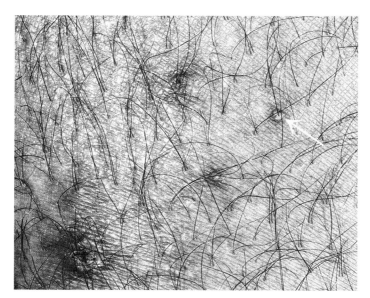

22–14. Bacterial folliculitis, showing hairs emerging from pustules (arrow). (*Courtesy of Richard P. Usatine, M.D.*)

Folliculitis

Folliculitis, by definition, originates in hair follicles. Bacterial folliculitis is often staphylococcal or streptococcal and can present in the pubic area, groin, buttocks, and perineum. Anecdotal experience in STD clinics suggest that the frequency of folliculitis may be rising in sexually active persons who shave the genital area, and some patients present with fear of herpes or other STD. The diagnostic hallmark of folliculitis is observation of a single hair emerging from some pustular lesions, helping distinguish the condition from herpes. In addition, folliculitis lesions generally are more widespread than those of genital herpes, and initial herpes generally involves the genitals per se rather than the pubic area, groin, or other hair-bearing areas.

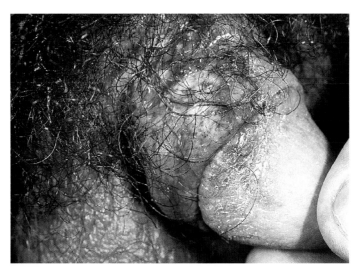

22–15. Pyoderma of the penis in a patient with scabies; *Staphylococcus aureus* was isolated.

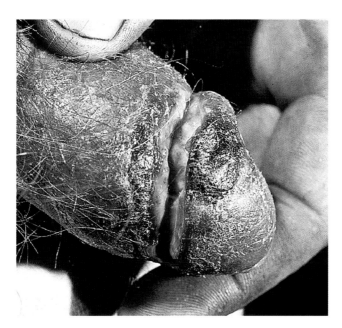

22–16. Penile pyoderma with necrotizing cellulitis in a man with secondary syphilis; *Staphylococcus aureus* and β-hemolytic *Streptococcus pyogenes* were isolated. This is the same patient whose secondary syphilis rash is shown in Fig. 5-21; he gave a history of a painless ulcer at the corona of the penis for 6 weeks before onset of penile pain and swelling.

Genital Pyoderma

Pyoderma and cellulitis of the genitals usually result from secondary infection of preexisting lesions. Scabies is a common predisposing factor among patients in STD clinics. Secondary bacterial infection of herpetic lesions or syphilitic chancres appears to be uncommon, although a chancre probably was the initial lesion in the patient in Fig. 22–16. Parenteral antibiotic therapy may be required for severe cases.

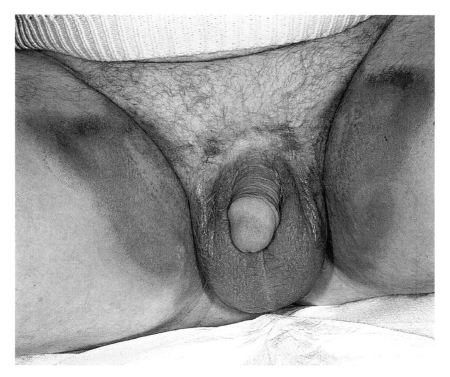

22–17. Erythrasma.

Erythrasma

Erythrasma is a superficial cutaneous infection, typically of the genitals, upper thighs, and crural folds, caused by *Corynebacterium minutissimum*. Most cases are less extensive than illustrated in Fig. 22–17. Chronic cases typically present with a copper-colored, red-brown rash with a raised border and fine scale. Bright coral-red fluorescence is seen under ultraviolet light (Wood's lamp). Erythrasma can be confused with tinea cruris (see Figs. 22–18 and 22–19), an important distinction as the treatments are different. Erythrasma is treated with oral clarithromycin or erythromycin; azithromycin probably would be effective but has not been studied.

Tinea Cruris

Tinea cruris is most common in men ("jock itch," Fig. 22–18) but is not rare in women (Fig. 22–19). It is caused by dermatophyte fungi, including *Trichophyton, Epidermophyton,* and *Microsporum* species. Tinea pedis (athlete's foot), caused by the same organisms, often is present simultaneously. Tinea cruris is characterized by an erythematous, papular, sometimes erosive dermatitis of the crural folds, inner thighs, or scrotum, with accentuated erythema and fine scale at the sharply demarcated border. The penis and labia usually are not involved. Tinea cruris can be confused with erythrasma (see Fig. 22–17) and other perigenital dermatoses, and the diagnosis can be difficult in dark-skinned patients, in whom erythema may be difficult to discern. Clinical diagnosis usually is reliable, but can be confirmed by scraping the advancing border and examining microscopically for fungal elements after digestion with 10% KOH. Topical imidazole creams such as miconazole (Micatin), ketoconazole (Nizoral), and others, as well as tolnaftate (Tinactin) and terbinafine (Lamisil) are effective; over-the-counter versions are readily available.

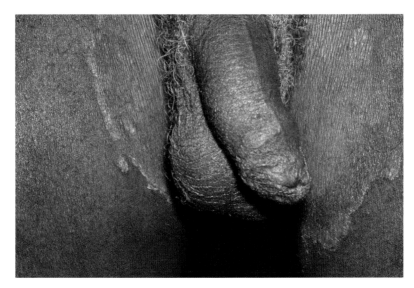

22–18. Tinea cruris, with annular scaling at the leading edge of the inflammatory lesion extending from the inguinal fold to the thighs. (*Reprinted with permission from Kelly AP, Taylor SC. Dermatology for Skin of Color. New York, NY: McGraw-Hill; 2009.*)

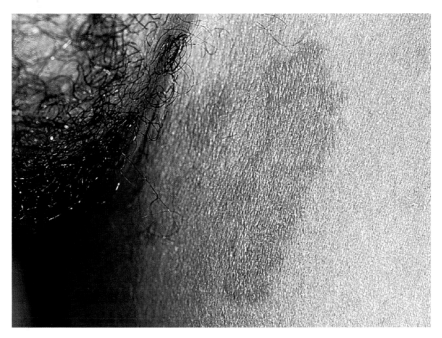

22–19. Tinea cruris. (*Courtesy of Philip Kirby, M.D.*)

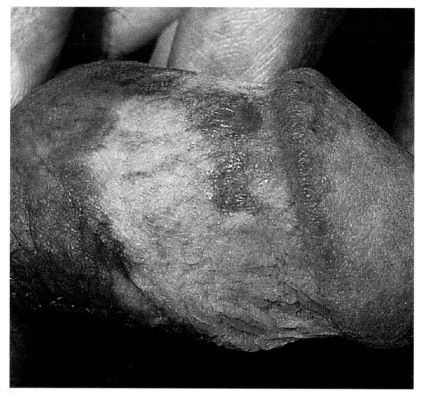

22–20. Vitiligo of the penis. (*Courtesy of Philip Kirby, M.D.*)

Vitiligo

Vitiligo is acquired cutaneous depigmentation resulting from loss of melanocytes, of probable autoimmune pathogenesis. Any area of the skin may be involved, but patients with genital involvement may present with concerns about STD. Although functionally harmless, vitiligo can be psychologically debilitating when it involves cosmetically sensitive areas, including the genitals. Some patients respond to treatment with topical or systemic corticosteroids, phototherapy, topical immunomodulators, or surgically using punch grafting of normally pigmented skin. Proper management requires dermatological expertise.

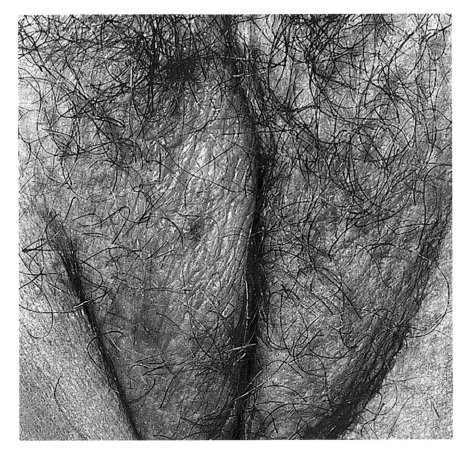

22–21. Lichen simplex chronicus of the vulva, with an ulcer caused by excoriation.

Lichen Simplex Chronicus

Lichen simplex chronicus usually presents as a solitary plaque, often quite large, with thickening of the skin and accentuated markings (lichenification), erythema, and sometimes excoriation. Involvement of the scrotum and labia majora is typical. The condition is more common in women than men and often accompanies other pruritic dermatoses, especially atopic dermatitis. The clinical manifestations primarily result from habitual scratching, which may be unconscious, and lesions are most common on the side of the dominant hand. Topical steroids and instruction to avoid scratching often are effective and dressings may help prevent unconscious scratching during sleep.

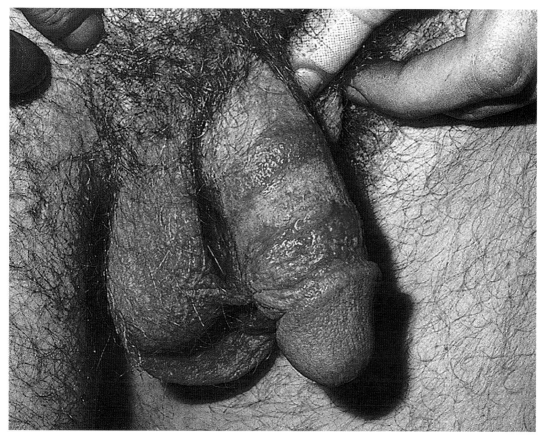

22–22. Contact dermatitis of the penis in a patient who was allergic to the adhesive tape of a bandage used to cover an episode of recurrent genital herpes; healing herpetic lesions are visible between the patches of acute dermatitis.

Contact Dermatitis

In its fully developed form, allergic contact dermatitis is characterized by vesicles or a denuded, weeping skin surface. History of exposure to potential irritants or allergens often is present. Removal of the inciting agent usually results in prompt resolution, although topical steroids may speed improvement.

Lichen Planus

Lichen planus is one of the most common genital dermatoses and is seen frequently in patients at risk for STD. The cause is unknown. The condition typically causes flat-topped papules with shiny surfaces, typically with a violaceous hue. Most lesions itch, but some are nonpruritic. Lichen nitidus (see Fig. 22–26) is a variation of lichen planus that presents with multiple small papules. Oral or genital mucosal lesions often are present, with lacy, serpiginous striae. When the lateral aspect of the tongue is involved, lichen planus can mimic HIV-related oral hairy leukoplakia (see Figs. 11-1c and 11-10). Most cases respond to topical corticosteroids.

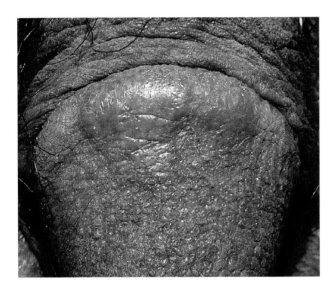

22–23. Lichen planus of the penis. (*Courtesy of Karl R. Beutner, M.D., Ph.D.*)

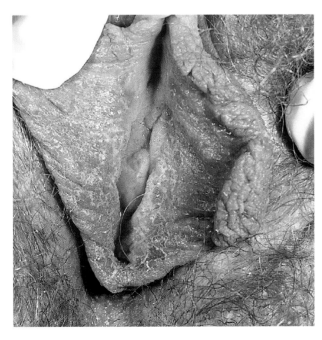

22–24. Lichen planus of the vaginal introitus, with faintly violaceous, serpiginous striations. Secondary lichenification of the labia minora also is present.

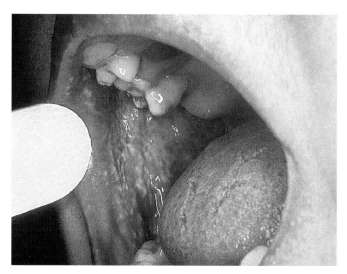

22–25. Lichen planus of the oral mucosa.

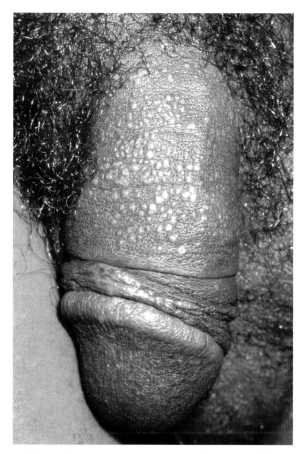

22–26. Lichen nitidus, generally considered a micropapular variant of lichen planus. A plaque of typical lichen planus is seen immediately proximal to the glans. (*Reprinted with permission from Wolff K, Johnson RA. Fitzpatrick's Color Atlas and Synopsis of Clinical Dermatology. 6th ed. New York, NY: McGraw-Hill; 2009.*)

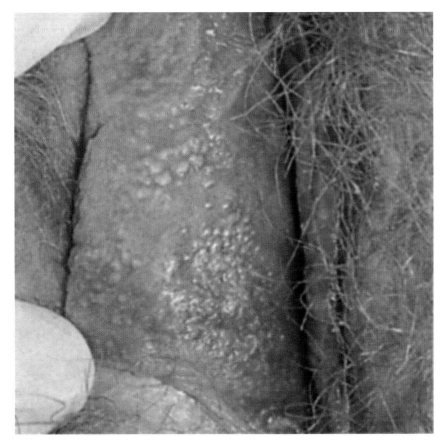

22–27. Fordyce spots of the penis. (*Reprinted with permission from Holmes KK, et al., eds. Sexually Transmitted Diseases. 4th ed. New York, NY: McGraw-Hill; 2008.*)

Fordyce Spots

Fordyce spots are prominent but anatomically normal sebaceous glands, most commonly observed in women on the inner aspect of the labia majora, but other sites, including the penis, can be involved. Individual papules typically are white or yellow and may appear more prominent in the presence of surrounding erythema due to other inflammatory conditions. For example, some women first notice Fordyce spots in the presence of vulvovaginal candidiasis. Anxious patients who first notice Fordyce spots may be concerned about STD. No treatment is required.

Pearly Penile Papules and Tyson Glands

Pearly penile papules are normal anatomic variants that appear as small (usually 0.5–1 mm) shiny papules of the penile corona, sometimes with filiform morphology. They are present in 10–20% of men, regardless of race or skin color, and are more common in circumcised than uncircumcised men.

"Tyson gland" has been used in reference to various normal anatomic variants of the penis. As usually used, Tyson glands—also known as preputial glands—are prominent, specialized sebaceous glands of the penile corona and inner surface of the foreskin. Sometimes they present as pairs located symmetrically on the ventral aspect of the penis immediately proximal to the glans; one, two, or sometimes three pairs may be present. Some affected men become concerned about STD when they first notice pearly penile papules or Tyson glands, or when they observe other men without them, and inexperienced clinicians may confuse them with genital warts, molluscum contagiosum, or other lesions.

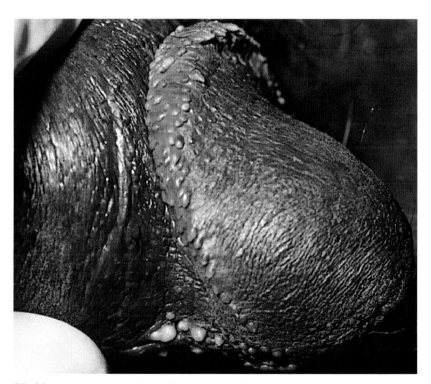

22–28. Pearly penile papules and Tyson glands. There are numerous pearly penile papules along the corona of the glans penis; the larger white papules on the ventral surface below the glans are Tyson glands. (*Courtesy of Philip Kirby, M.D.*)

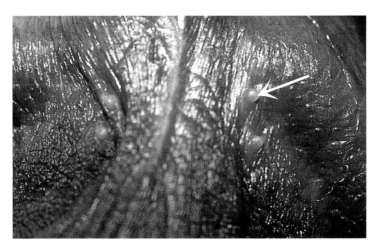

22–29. Four Tyson glands, two on each side of the meatus; one gland is denoted by the white arrow. (*Courtesy of Karl R. Beutner, M.D., Ph.D.*)

Vestibular Papillomatosis

Vestibular papillomatosis is considered the female counterpart of pearly penile papules and typically presents with multiple soft papules of the vaginal introitus or labia minora, usually symmetrically distributed. The condition may be confused with genital warts by both patients and providers. As for pearly penile papules, Tyson glands, and Fordyce spots, vestibular papillomatosis is a normal anatomic variant.

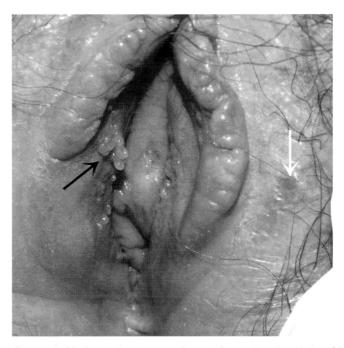

22–30. Vestibular papillomatosis (black arrow); compare with genital warts (see Figs. 8–1 and 8–4) and pearly penile papules of the penis (see Fig. 22–28). The patient complained of vulvar pruritus and has a lesion consistent with recurrent genital herpes (white arrow). (*Courtesy of Chih-Chieh Chan, M.D. and Hisen-Ching Chiu, M.D.; reprinted with permission from Chan C-C, Chiu H-C. Vestibular papillomatosis. N Engl J Med. 2008;358:1495.*)

SUGGESTED READING

Edwards L, Lynch PJ. *Genital Dermatology Atlas.* 2nd ed. Philadelphia, PA: Wolters Kluwer | Lippincott Williams & Wilkins; 2011 (336 pp). *An extensively illustrated atlas and text of dermatoses that commonly affect the genitals.*

Kelly AP, Taylor SC. *Dermatology for Skin of Color.* New York, NY: McGraw-Hill; 2009 (722 pp). *An especially useful clinical reference when dark-skinned patients present with dermatological complaints.*

Torgerson RR, Edwards L. Genital dermatoses. Chapter 64 in Holmes KK et al., eds. *Sexually Transmitted Diseases.* 4th ed. New York, NY: McGraw-Hill; 2008:1209-26. *Review of common conditions that may be seen by clinicians providing STD services.*

Usatine RP, et al (eds). *The Color Atlas of Family Medicine.* New York, NY: Mc-Graw-Hill; 2009 (1095 pp). *Comprehensive illustrations and review of common dermatologic conditions for the non-specialist, as well as cutaneous manifestations of systemic disease and non-dermatologic conditions.*

Wolff K, Johnson RA. *Fitzpatrick's Color Atlas and Synopsis of Clinical Dermatology.* 6th ed. New York, NY: McGraw-Hill; 2009 (1114 pp). *A comprehensive, extensively illustrated review of dermatologic conditions, with format and approach similar to this book.*

Appendix

Medical and Sexual History, Physical Examination, and Laboratory Evaluation of STD Patients

This outline is derived from the clinical record of the Public Health—Seattle & King County STD Clinic.* All elements can be expressed in check-off format or with numerical entries. In the author's clinic, separate male and female records are printed on three pages, with sufficient space for expanded written findings.

HISTORY

Reason(s) for Visit

- Symptoms
- STD exposure (specify)
- Positive STD test (specify)
- No symptoms; request for STD screening
- HIV test
- Referral (specify source)

---

* Clinicians and health care agencies are invited to adopt this outline for clinical use, without regard to copyright or other restrictions. Copies of the STD medical record itself can be obtained from the author.

Symptoms[†]

Males

- Urethral symptoms
  - Discharge
  - Dysuria
  - Urinary urgency or frequency
  - Altered urine flow
  - Other
- Genital lesion(s) or rash
- Nongenital skin rash
- Anorectal symptoms
  - Pain, pruritus
  - Lesion(s)
  - Discharge, including pus or mucus observed on feces
  - Bleeding
  - Other (tenesmus, diarrhea, constipation, etc.)
- Testicular symptoms
  - Pain
  - Swelling
  - Other
- Oral or pharyngeal symptoms
  - Lesions/sores
  - Sore throat
  - Other
- Systemic symptoms, e.g., fever, malaise, etc.
- Swelling or pain that suggests lymphadenopathy (neck, armpits, groin, etc.)
- Other (specify)

Females

- Vulvovaginal symptoms
  - Abnormal or increased vaginal discharge
  - Malodor (characterize)

[†] Symptoms are denoted with check boxes, followed by space to indicate duration in days.

- ○ Pruritus
- ○ External dysuria[‡]
- ○ Other (specify)
- Urinary symptoms
  - ○ Internal dysuria[‡]
  - ○ Urgency, frequency
  - ○ Other (specify)
- Genital lesion(s) or rash
- Abdominal or pelvic pain
- Abnormal vaginal bleeding
  - ○ Amount
  - ○ Frequency
  - ○ Timing with respect to menstruation
  - ○ Circumstances (e.g., post-coital)
- Nongenital skin rash
- Anorectal symptoms
  - ○ Pain, pruritus
  - ○ Lesion(s)
  - ○ Discharge, including pus or mucus observed on feces
  - ○ Bleeding
  - ○ Other, specify (tenesmus, diarrhea, constipation, etc.)
- Oral or pharyngeal symptoms
  - ○ Lesions/sores
  - ○ Sore throat
  - ○ Other
- Systemic symptoms, e.g., fever, malaise, etc.
- Swelling or pain that suggests lymphadenopathy (neck, armpits, groin, etc.)
- Other (specify)

Drugs and Medications

- Drug allergies
- Antibiotics and antiviral drugs in past month

[‡] External dysuria denotes painful urination from contact of urine with introitus or labia. Internal dysuria means urethral or bladder pain during urination.

Illicit drug use (ever, current, most recent; association with sexual risks)

Alcohol use and abuse (ever, current, most recent; association with sexual risks)

HIV Status and Risks

HIV status

If positive:

- Date of diagnosis
- Current HIV health care
- Current antiretroviral therapy
- HIV viral load
- CD4+ cell count
- Risk of transmission:
  - Sexual activity
  - HIV status of current sex partner(s)
  - Condom use
  - Drug use with shared injection equipment

If negative or unknown:

- Date of last negative test
- Risk Assessment (Ever, Past 12 months, Most Recent)
  - For males: Sex with other men
  - For females: Sex with MSM
  - Sex with HIV-infected person
  - Sex with injection drug user
  - Injection drug use
  - Commercial sex
  - Multiple (e.g., ≥4) opposite sex partners in past year
  - Other risk (specify)
  - None of the above

Sexual History

- Number of sex partners in past year
  - Opposite sex
  - Same sex
  - Transgender

- Sexual exposures (elicited separately for opposite-sex and same-sex partners)

  ○ Number of partners, past 2 months and 12 months

  ○ Time since last sex with regular sex partner

  ○ Time since first sex with a new partner

  ○ Partners believed to have other recent sex partners

  ○ Anatomic sites exposed in past 2 months (penis, vagina, rectum, mouth/throat)

  ○ Condom use during most recent penile-insertive sex

- For MSM

  ○ Number of anonymous (i.e., unidentifiable) partners in past 2 months

  ○ Frequency of condom use in past 2 months (recorded separately for anal insertive and anal receptive intercourse)

Past STD

For each condition, record whether past infection ever (yes/no). If yes, record number of episodes and date or time since most recent episode.

- Chlamydia

- Gonorrhea

- Syphilis

  ○ Stage

  ○ Treatment

  ○ Follow-up

- Genital herpes

  ○ Initial infection

  ○ Recurrent outbreaks (frequency, most recent)

  ○ Virus type (HSV-1, HSV-2, unknown)

- Human papillomavirus infection

  ○ Genital warts

  ○ Anal or rectal warts

  ○ Other external genital lesions (e.g., PIN, VIN, VaIN)

  ○ Abnormal Pap smear (women only; stage, treatment, year)

- Nongonococcal urethritis (NGU) (men only)

- Cervical and vaginal infections (women only)

  ○ Mucopurulent cervicitis (MPC)

  ○ Trichomoniasis

- ○ Bacterial vaginosis
- ○ Yeast vulvovaginitis
- Pelvic inflammatory disease (women only)
- Viral hepatitis (A, B, C)
- Other STD (specify)

STD Immunizations

- Human papillomavirus vaccine (yes, no, uncertain)

If yes:

- ○ Vaccine type (bivalent, quadrivalent)
- ○ Number of doses
- ○ Date of last dose
- Hepatitis B vaccine (yes, no, uncertain)

If yes:

- ○ Number of doses
- ○ Date of last dose

Obstetric and Gynecologic History (Women)

- Date of last normal menstrual period
- Pregnancy
  - ○ Gravidity
  - ○ Parity
  - ○ Abortion(s), spontaneous
  - ○ Abortion(s), induced
- Most recent cervical cytology (date, result)
- Douching in past year (yes/no)
- Currently attempting to conceive or hoping to become pregnant (yes/no)
- Contraceptive method(s) in past 2 months
  - ○ None
  - ○ Oral
  - ○ Other hormonal contraception (ring, patch, implant, injection: specify)
  - ○ Intrauterine device (IUD)
  - ○ Condoms; with or without spermicide
  - ○ Surgical sterilization: Tubal ligation, hysterectomy
  - ○ Partner vasectomy or sterile

PHYSICAL EXAMINATION

Males

- General appearance
- Skin (examine all exposed skin surfaces)
- Mouth and throat
- Circumcision status
- Urethral meatus and discharge
    - Meatal erythema, edema
    - Discharge amount: None, scant, moderate (easily expressed), large (spontaneous)
    - Character: Clear, mucopurulent, purulent
- Genital lesions
    - (vesicle, pustule, papule, etc.)
    - Location(s)
    - Number, size, clustering
- Scrotal/testicular palpation (size, consistency, mass, tenderness, testicular elevation)
- Lymphadenopathy (consistency, size, tenderness, fluctuance, overlying erythema)
    - Inguinal (unilateral, bilateral)
    - Other locations (specify)
- Anorectal examination if symptomatic or history of anal exposure
    - Visual inspection of anus, perineum
    - Anoscopy (selected patients)

Females

- General appearance
- Skin (examine all exposed skin surfaces)
- Mouth and throat
- Vulva, labia, introitus, perineum
- Genital lesions
    - (vesicle, pustule, papule, etc.)
    - Location(s)
    - Number, size, clustering
- Vagina and vaginal secretions
    - Amount: None, scant, moderate, large
    - Color: White or gray, yellow/purulent, brown, sanguinous
    - Character: Floccular, homogenous, adherent, plaques or clumps

- Cervix
  - Lesions
  - Ectopy (extent, edema)
  - Swab-induced endocervical bleeding ("Friability")
  - Discharge (amount, color, character)
- Bimanual pelvic examination
  - Cervical motion tenderness
  - Uterine fundus (size, form, tenderness)
  - Adnexal tenderness
  - Adnexal or other pelvic mass
- Lymphadenopathy (consistency, size, tenderness, fluctuance, overlying erythema)
  - Inguinal (unilateral, bilateral)
  - Other locations (specify)
- Anorectal examination if symptomatic or history of anal exposure
  - Visual inspection of anus, perineum
  - Anoscopy (selected patients)

LABORATORY TESTS†

Microscopy, Cytology, and Rapid Tests

- Gram-stained smear (cervix, or specify other site)
- Vaginal fluid tests
  - Wet-mount microscopy for clue cells, trichomonads (saline), fungi (10% KOH)
  - pH
  - Amine odor test (KOH "sniff") test
- Darkfield microscopy (in settings where early syphilis is commonly diagnosed)
- Rapid plasma reagin (or other rapid syphilis serology)
- Leukocyte esterase
- Urinalysis (leukocyte esterase, chemistry dipstick, dipstick, microscopy)
- Cervical cytology (Pap smear)
  - HPV NAAT

---

† Most of the tests listed should be readily available in STD clinics and other settings frequently attended by patients with STD or at risk. However, even STD clinics may find it impractical to offer routine testing for rare conditions, such as tests for *H. ducreyi* in settings where chancroid is absent or rare. Darkfield microscopy is optional in settings where syphilis is rare, and not all clinics require both point-of-care and laboratory-based HIV antibody tests. The selection of tests for routine screening or diagnosis varies with patients' symptoms, exposure history, epidemiologic circumstances, the local prevalence and incidence of various STDs, and specific assays available in local or regional laboratories. See Chap. 1 for recommendations for routine STD assessment in most primary care settings.

- Microscopy of skin scrapings for scabies
- Rapid pregnancy testing

Microbiologic and Virologic Tests

- *Neisseria gonorrhoeae* NAAT or culture: specify sites or specimens (cervix, vaginal swab, urine, rectum, pharynx)
- *Chlamydia trachomatis* NAAT: specify sites or specimens (cervix, vaginal swab, urine, rectum)
- Herpes simplex virus NAAT or culture, including determination of virus type (specify sites or specimens)
- *Haemophilus ducreyi* culture or NAAT
- *Trichomonas vaginalis:* culture or NAAT
- Urine culture for uropathogens
- Culture or NAAT for cutaneous bacterial pathogens, e.g., *Staphylococcus*, *Streptococcus* (specify sites or specimens)

Blood Tests

- Syphilis serology
  - Nontreponemal reaginic test, e.g., RPR, VDRL, or TRUST (qualitative and quantitative)
  - *Treponema pallidum*-specific test, e.g., enzyme immunoassay (EIA) or traditional treponemal test such as *T. pallidum* particle agglutination test (TPPA)
- HIV diagnostics
  - Laboratory-based antibody test, e.g., EIA
  - Combination HIV antibody and p24 antigen assay
  - Rapid (point-of-care) antibody test
  - HIV Western blot
  - HIV virologic tests, e.g., NAAT for HIV RNA, p24 antigen
- HSV type-specific serological test (antibody to HSV-1 and HSV-2)
- Viral hepatitis serology
  - Hepatitis A virus (HAV) antibody
  - Hepatitis B virus (HBV): Hepatitis B surface antigen (HBsAg), antibody to surface antigen (HBsAb), antibody to core antigen (HBcAb)
  - Hepatitis C virus (HCV) antibody

Index

Page numbers referencing figures are followed by a *f* and page numbers referencing tables are followed by a *t*